T0131620

Your Body
Is Not
Your Enemy

A New Guide to Getting Over Your Self
and Enjoying Optimal Health

JEFF WOITON

BALBOA.
PRESS

A DIVISION OF HAY HOUSE

Balboa Press books may be ordered through booksellers or by contacting:

Balboa Press
A Division of Hay House
1663 Liberty Drive
Bloomington, IN 47403
www.balboapress.com
1 (877) 407-4847

Because of the dynamic nature of the Internet, any web addresses or
links contained in this book may have changed since publication and
may no longer be valid. The views expressed in this work are solely those
of the author and do not necessarily reflect the views of the publisher,
and the publisher hereby disclaims any responsibility for them.

The contents of this book and any related materials, including cited
references, are for informational purposes only and are not intended to be a
substitute for professional medical advice, diagnosis, or treatment. Always
seek the advice of your physician or other qualified health provider with
any questions you may have regarding a specific medical condition.

Any people depicted in stock imagery provided by Thinkstock are
models, and such images are being used for illustrative purposes only.
Certain stock imagery © Thinkstock.

Print information available on the last page.

ISBN: 978-1-5043-3177-7 (sc)
ISBN: 978-1-5043-3179-1 (hc)
ISBN: 978-1-5043-3178-4 (e)

Library of Congress Control Number: 2015906294

Balboa Press rev. date: 06/23/2015

This book is dedicated to the millions of people
who have chosen to get over their selves
and to do the hard work it takes
to enjoy optimal health
using nothing more than
natural food and natural remedies.

They may be unknown to me,
but they have been my greatest inspiration.
I hope they will inspire you to do the same.

Contents

Preface

Many of the people I have met in the healing arts first came from a place of serious illness, either as their own experience or with a loved one, coupled with a hard-earned frustration at the weaknesses of our current medical system. Their condition sent them to varying levels of self-study into healing their condition and uncovering a wide spectrum of advice that might end up being helpful or harmful or somewhere in between. Such a spectrum is easily found on the Internet, which offers a great amount of helpful information along with loads and loads of useless junk, and it's difficult for the layperson to discern at which end of that spectrum they're looking. The signal-to-noise ratio is high, and I'm sure there are people who have inflicted significant harm as a result of trying something they read online that sounded good at the time. This book was never intended to try and be all things to all people, and I'm sure that there are portions that will leave you feeling left out while other parts may strike a familiar chord. I urge you to take what you want from this book, do your own research to learn more, and, if necessary, seek the help of a qualified healthcare practitioner whose opinion you trust.

Here's my story: I come from a family of five boys. My father was a US Army officer, so we moved around a lot. My mother did all she could to keep the appetites of five hungry boys satiated. Leftovers were uncommon; she would make a huge pot of soup or stew or spaghetti and there would be none left by the time the first of us got up from the table. I carried those eating habits into my adult life, and for the most part I felt well, although as I got older my weight slowly began to increase and I started having occasional and inexplicable bouts of intestinal illness. When I joined the US Navy at age eighteen, I weighed a hundred and thirty-nine pounds at six feet tall. Despite my diet and eating habits, I was always a skinny kid. By the time I left the Navy, I was probably around a hundred and seventy-five, but that only mildly discouraged me. Overall, I felt fine and thought that a little weight gain was an appropriate part of adulthood.

A few years later, I began to have episodes of stabbing intestinal pain coupled with diarrhea that would last for two weeks or more. It became difficult to get ready for work when I would need to go to the bathroom ten or twelve times just during the time it took me to get showered and dressed. Then, once I was at work, I was often interrupted by sharp abdominal pains and a sudden urge to go to the toilet. I remember having such an attack as I was training about a dozen newly-hired employees. I suddenly left the topic at hand for them to discuss amongst themselves as I dashed down several hallways to get to the men's room, which was never located close enough. I'm glad to say I never had a public accident, but knowing that it could happen at almost any time and the disgusting feeling of potential filthiness it left me with greatly lowered my mood.

Then my symptoms would gradually subside, and I thought little more of it except for the lucky feeling that I'd returned to normal for a while. I was likely still undergoing a mild form of intestinal perforation, and I might feel OK for even a few years, when suddenly something would trigger those same symptoms and the whole process would start over again.

Let's fast-forward a few decades. In 2008, my wife notified me rather abruptly that she wanted a divorce so she could move to Florida and be with an old high school boyfriend. Ouch! So I did what seemed like the only sensible thing to do, which was to try to run away from my problems. I had an opportunity to manage a café on the island of Utila, one of the Bay Islands of Honduras in the Caribbean. There were many wonderful things I had gotten out of that experience, including getting my Advanced Open Water SCUBA certificate and dramatically improving my knowledge of kitchen Spanish (the phrase, "¿Como se dice?" proved invaluable here), but eventually it became a rather costly lark and I longed to return to my adopted hometown of Seattle. Paradise is overrated.

Once back in Seattle, with the divorce settlement finalized and flush with cash after selling my portion of a very nice house we had together, I moved into a small apartment and pondered my next move. I had tried a few things, even attempting to get my old job back, but nothing stuck. Then I began to notice those dreaded symptoms returning once again. I soon found myself doubled over in pain and visiting the bathroom several times a day, all day long. I began to lose all interest in food, even though I had always loved preparing and cooking and eating food. I would go to the grocery store and find nothing that interested me. I lost weight at an alarming rate - over forty-five pounds in just six weeks. I slept much of the day, when I wasn't using the bathroom or hating food, and eventually found that had gotten so weak I would get winded just walking a few yards. My voice became thin and high-pitched, my hands trembled, and I was severely disoriented and depressed and isolating myself inside my little apartment. I wondered to myself if I had come down with a serious illness, and even thought whether this was how my life was meant to end. I felt indifferent to my own existence, but as you can tell I ultimately thought better of that notion. I was going out of control in a terrible spiral that nearly led me to a grim end.

Nothing was working, and I knew my life was falling apart. I didn't have a job, and therefore didn't have health insurance, so in my depressed state I felt that I was, as they say in the Navy, screwed without a kiss. But one evening, before I went to bed, I made the decision that I would take action and do something. I knew that my options were running out, and I would need to act and act fast. I got out a sticky note and wrote this on it:

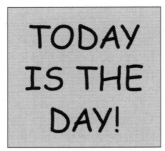

I meant this as a reminder to myself so that, when I woke up, that day would be the day that I would somehow manage the strength to do something about my prematurely declining health. I had stuck the note on the wall in the hallway outside my bedroom door so that if and when I got up the next morning I would see it and maybe - just maybe - consider doing something about my condition. I knew I needed to do something and, since I have no immediate family living nearby, I would have to rely on myself and my own inner strength to get started and to follow through on this. My choices were narrowed down to either doing something, or slowly dying alone in an apartment with no one around. I chose to help myself.

I had heard about a clinic in town that took cases from low-income patients with inadequate or no insurance. I got bathed and shaved and dressed, looking presentable for the first time in several days, and wrote down a list of every symptom I was feeling at the time. I drove a short distance to the clinic, filled in a new patient form, and waited my turn to be seen. I was told by the person at the front desk that, as a new patient, it would be two to three weeks before I could get in to see a doctor. I hope I have presented the state of my health during that time well enough by now to impress upon you that two to three weeks would not be manageable. I was in severe pain, weak as a kitten, and might actually be dying. I thanked them for the brief chat and left without making an appointment.

While I was waiting, I considered what other options I might have. Since I had been in the Navy, I wondered if the VA hospital might be something to look into. There were rumors and stories of neglect and abuse and poor management throughout the VA healthcare system, but by that point I felt I had nothing to lose. I found where the main facility in Seattle was located, and since it was just across town I sallied forth. Once there, I went to the registration desk and asked how I could get treatment. The young lady at the desk, a veteran herself, looked me up by name and Social Security number and quickly found that I had indeed served and was honorably discharged, and so, yes, I was eligible for benefits. Then she asked me if I would like to be seen today. My response was weak but ecstatic: "Really? You mean I can see a doctor today?" Her affirmative answer gave me instant relief, and I was directed to Urgent Care.

Once I got in to see the Urgent Care physician, I handed him my symptom list and sheepishly bleated something like, "Fix me." I'm sure that the doctor must have felt somewhat daunted and perplexed, but he systematically made his way through my list and conducted a brief triage of what I'd presented to him. In the next few days I was assigned to a primary care physician who tried various protocols to deal with the handful of symptoms I'd come in with. I was feeling jim-dandy about myself for a few days at having taken a stand for my own health, but I still had the symptoms and the pain. I began to notice that I wasn't seeing much improvement, and finally I just went back to the VA hospital without an appointment, prepared only with a determination to wait until they could fit me in. After a couple of hours, I got the chance to see my doctor. I told her that I was still suffering from acute pain and diarrhea and most of the other symptoms, and her response was just this: "I'm admitting you."

I got to spend five days as a patient at the VA Hospital. They weren't sure what to do with me, but they were pretty sure I was a sick man. I had a great number of good friends who came to visit me, which was immeasurable in raising my spirits. Someone who I hardly knew brought me flowers. My friend David Huber, a busy downtown attorney, was at my bedside within an hour after he heard I was in the hospital, having apparently dropped everything he was doing to come to my bedside. Hospitals have a way of making healthy people feel uncomfortable, and I'm sure many of the people who visited me may have felt a little off, but seeing them all did wonders for my recovery.

When I was released, I felt like I was starting to get better. The doctor who'd performed a colonoscopy described my intestines as being like "the inside of a burned-out building" because of all the inflammation he saw. They started me on Remicade (infliximab), which, I was told, is normally given to organ transplant patients to lower their immune system and thus to prevent them from rejecting the donor organ. I went in dutifully every eight weeks for over a year as they hooked up an IV line into the back of my hand and pumped Remicade into my system, never thinking that they should be supporting my immune system rather than weakening it.

The healing effects of Remicade were mostly rather subtle, and near the end of each eight-week period, just before it was time to go in again, I would slowly start to feel the return of some of the symptoms I'd been feeling before. I also read up on Remicade and found these as possible side effects:

- serious and sometimes fatal blood disorders
- serious infections
- lymphoma and solid tissue cancers
- reports of serious liver injury
- reactivation of hepatitis B
- reactivation of tuberculosis

- lethal hepatosplenic T-cell lymphoma
- drug-induced lupus
- demyelinating central nervous system disorders
- psoriasis and psoriasiform skin lesions
- new-onset vitiligo

So – Remicade could give me cancer, death, and vitiligo. Sure, the chances might be slim, but I came to realize, through both research and my own logical deductions, that switching my diet to just whole, natural foods might be a better choice. I was not aware that food in any combination or quantity could give me any of the above symptoms. I finally decided that I would really and truly take charge of my own health, and I eventually had the "break-up conversation" with my gastroenterologist. I told him I no longer wanted to take the prescribed medication, and, as the patient, I felt I had every right to choose this for myself. His response was that, if I were to have another outbreak, my body will have developed antigens that would render Remicade ineffective. I confirmed with him that all I needed to do was avoid having any further outbreaks. We agreed to call it a draw, and I stopped going in to the IV clinic every eight weeks.

Since I was eating better food, I started feeling better and the symptoms began to abate. After my hospital stay I had managed to gain back all the weight I'd lost and then some, from a low of about 172 to over 250. I had gone on some wrong pathways, nutritionally speaking, but once I had switched my diet back to whole natural foods, including cutting out sugar, I started losing weight at the more reasonable pace of about five pounds a month.

Around the same time, I became aware of a program, offered through a local community college and hosted by the Nutritional Therapy Association, to become certified as a Nutritional Therapy Practitioner. I felt that the program would help me to understand more about how people can find themselves in a condition similar to mine, and how I could help them find their back way out of it as I had done. The tuition got paid, the books arrived, and I was a student once again.

At the risk of making a crass and brazen plug, I found the NTA's curriculum to be intensive and well planned. I studied the basics of digestion and, in the process, overcame my own tendency to be grossed out by it all, and so I delved further into topics such as blood sugar regulation, fatty acid and mineral balance, endocrinology, and the roles of individual vitamins and amino acids. This was mostly an online course, but we would meet as a class once a semester for lectures, testing, and practical exercises. We learned how to conduct clinical interviews, perform functional evaluations, and carry out Lingual-Neural Testing. The class was about ninety percent women, with maybe five or six male students. I wondered whether this data point made any difference, and it really doesn't. Rather, it opened me up to what I felt was my true calling-within-a-calling: that I could focus on the health issues of men over age forty.

So here I am, some time later and with a burgeoning practice in the healing arts. I see clients from all walks of life and bearing the full gamut of conditions. I found myself telling them some of the same things over and over again, and so this book is a way of sharing my story and some of the general concepts of proper health with a wider audience. I'll mention more about the concept of bioindividuality later on in the book, but I'd like it to be clear that the statements I make here are merely my best suggestions for you. In order to truly bring yourself to the best possible state of health, it's up to you to seek out the help of a nutritional therapist or anyone else who can help you work with and within your unique and specific condition.

I use the terms 'yourself' and 'your self' differently in this book, and it's intentional and within the context of the statement being made. I use 'yourself' in the common manner and 'your self' to underscore the awareness of you and who you are. I love words, and I intend to use plenty of them here. When I was a young reader I would make the effort to look up new words and find out what they mean, their etymology, and how I can incorporate them into my everyday speech. I may explain the meanings of some of the bigger words I use here, and if I do not, then I urge you to follow my habit of looking them up and finding out their meanings for yourself. In this day and age, the Internet is your friend.

I also realize that there's probably a lot I'm leaving out here. If you're a gastroenterologist, for example, you're probably going to roll your eyes at my glossed-over description of the digestive process. So go ahead, roll them now and get it out of the way, and then read on anyhow. It's possible that you might glean something that they never taught you in med school, or perhaps you'll see the same thing presented in a new light. Let your self be open to getting new information, or to being reacquainted with something familiar said in a different voice. Take what you want and leave the rest.

It's also true that this book holds a rather U.S.-centric view of food policy. This is consistent with my understanding that Americans have some of the poorest diets of the industrialized world, and, as such, have some of the most dramatic self-inflicted health issues imaginable. If you are in another country as you read this and are thinking to yourself, "Oh, those poor Americans," I would not take issue with that sentiment.

Acknowledgements

I always wanted to write a book, and so I have, but this effort could not have transformed from possibility to reality without the kind assistance from some truly incredible people in my life.

First and foremost, Emmett Pritchard is not a stand-up guy, he is *the* stand-up guy. He and Sophie Koltchak Pritchard were always there for me when I needed a friend the most.

NTA lead instructor John Tjenos taught me much of the hands-on work that a Nutritional Therapist does and, from many years of experience, his knowledge of his craft is profound. Furthermore, I want to thank Gray Graham for creating the Nutritional Therapy Association, and Toni Blanton, of the NTA, for her kind assistance with my coursework.

My late parents, J.B. and Jan Woiton, never told me that cooking is just for girls, though I suppose that's how it goes in a family of all boys. Everyone eats, and so everyone should know how to cook. Some people think that cooking is difficult; Mom and Dad both showed me how easy and fun it can be.

As a practitioner of Dahn Body and Brain Education, I finally attained the clarity of mental focus to begin and complete this book. Dahn has helped me to sincerely believe that I can go on to do great things. Instrumental in getting me from there to here are Master Hyeran Ihm, Master Danielle Gaudette, and Master Gi Juek, among so many others. And it was from a lecture by Master Sayong Kim, during a meditation retreat he'd led at Mago Garden Retreat Center near Sedona, that I got the inspiration for the title of this book. Furthermore, I want to acknowledge Ilchi Lee Sunsanim for his profound inspiration and spiritual guidance.

Nancy Nickerson is office manager in the Health Promotion and Wellness Department at Illinois State University, and her help in guiding me through the hitherto unknown process of writing and editing a book is as immeasurable as her wit and charm. Jamie Wheeler is a professor of English and lead editor at eNotes.com to whom I've gone far too many times for random questions about writing style. Jory Kahn, a certified Feldenkrais practitioner and avid surf kayaker who plays a mean guitar, also lent tremendous support to the editing effort.

Lastly, I would not have been able to publish this book at all without the kind generosity of all of the people who contributed to my Kickstarter project and other fundraising campaigns. I was truly amazed at how my friends rallied around my dream to make this book happen, and there were many people whom I hadn't heard from in years who had pledged goodly sums towards my campaign. I greatly appreciate your generous support.

David Bristol	Hyeran Ihm
Penny Browder	Brandon Jemeyson
Dion Casto	Sean Jones
Allen Cent	Tracy Kish
Ginger Chaffin	John Kohlsaat
Brent Cleary	Paul Larsen
Eddie Cordero	Martin Lockwood
Peter Drury	Kelly McCormick
Kimberley Edmondson	Mack McCoy
Dave and Vicki Field	Michael Medina
Tim Garner	Kirk Mellendorf
Elma Garza	Susan J. Michael
Ken Grainger	Tom and Joanna Nelson
Jan Hansen	Nancy Nickerson
Burr Hitchcock	Karen Pauley

Olemara Peters
Pam Pollock
Brenda Pryor
Ames Reinhold
Michele Riggio
Brianna Sieberg
Maureen Shallit
Agen Schmitz
John Slate

Laura Diane Smith
Ngaire Taylor
Chi Vu
Norma Whatcott
Linda Wiley
James Woiton
Jerry Woiton
Joel Woiton and Lisa Casto
John and DeeAnna Woiton

SECTION I

Health

"Perhaps all the dragons in our lives are princesses who are only waiting to see us act, just once, with beauty and courage. Perhaps everything that frightens us is, in its deepest essence, something helpless that wants our love."
                                        Rainer Maria Rilke

The human body is a wonderful machine that is capable of undergoing severe punishment, grievous damage, and debilitating illness, and then working hard toward recovery in an attempt to return itself to optimal health. We may try to attain some level of equilibrium consciously, but our bodies tirelessly work to restore balance within our system as a whole. Your body is doing the best that it can to try and maintain order, based on what we give it to work with. This order is known as homeostasis, and it's the balance that we all strive for, whether we are aware that it's happening or not. No matter what we do to ourselves, from sports injuries to poor eating habits, your body will try to recover from what you've managed to do to it. Life happens, though, and through our own experiences and the choices we make, we either steer ourselves toward better health or away from it. We usually seek out healthy choices, we try our best, but often something comes up that causes us to want to eat something we know we shouldn't.

Sometimes I slip into old habits and eat something that I know isn't the best choice for me. It happens, and when it does, I simply try to stop what I'm doing, put it away (after the initial rush of guilty pleasure has subsided), and go back to my diet of nutrient-dense properly prepared whole and natural foods. Even the most conscientious of us fall into moments of food relapse, backsliding into a brief lack of firm control.

But the human body is such a truly astounding creation, capable of healing and repairing itself when occasional slip-ups come into our lives. We are all highly developed organisms of astonishing innate intelligence that can regulate all of the body's functions so that we don't have to think too much about, for example, our hypothalamus as it signals our adrenal glands to release cortisol to regulate our blood sugar. It just happens, and by making a few changes in our eating habits, we can ensure that those signals keep happening at the right time and for the right reasons.

If you cut yourself, your blood will quickly coagulate and stop itself from bleeding more than you have to. A scab begins to form, which will ultimately fall off as the skin grows itself back together. Within a short time, there will be little evidence of your wound, and your body has restored itself back to a reasonable state of repaired function.

So it is with many of your organs. Your liver can completely regenerate new cells from damaged ones in as little as three to four days (in a process called compensatory hypertrophy). Blood vessels that have collapsed or constricted can re-route the flow of blood to nearby arteries. You shed skin cells and hairs and intestinal cells at the rate of millions per day, only to be replaced by healthy new cells in a never-ending parade. Your lungs are also self-cleaning and self-healing; smokers who quit have the same chance of contracting lung cancer as non-smokers within just a few years.

If you find yourself in a state of poor health, you can rebuild yourself through a rigorous protocol of swapping junk food for real food. It's as simple as that, and as complex as the seven-plus billion individuals that make up this planet. Learning what is right for your body and your condition is where it all starts.

How Health Happens

One holistic approach is to look at how health happens in six distinct stages: molecules, cells, tissues, organs, systems, and the organism as a whole. If we are taking in all the proper molecules – meaning the proper minerals, vitamins, amino acids, fatty acids, polysaccharides, and so on – each of them will do their part to support the cell structures of various tissues, which will support the organs that comprise our various systems and ultimately lead to a happy and healthy organism. Conversely, if the cells do not get all the right kinds of molecules that they need to grow and flourish, there will be defects in the tissue structures that can contribute to the failure of the organ, a breakdown of the system, or, as the rate of tissue degeneration exceeds the body's rate of repair, ultimately bring about the death of the organism.

It sounds scary, but it happens every day. Even the healthiest of us are at some stage of this process at any given moment, fluctuating up or down on the scale of optimal health. Though the human body is amazingly strong and resilient, as I've mentioned before, our bodies are ultimately self-destructing machines, and life is a condition from which no one escapes. I look upon optimal health as a process, not an event. It's not like you can work your way to optimal health, hands in the air as you victoriously cross the finish line, breaking the tape with your chest and high-fiving everyone in sight because you're now at optimal health. It's likely that you may never achieve what is considered "optimal" health

The Downward Spiral of Cells

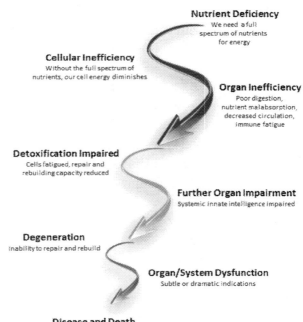

Nutrient Deficiency
We need a full
spectrum of nutrients
for energy

Cellular Inefficiency
Without the full spectrum of
nutrients, our cell energy diminishes

Organ Inefficiency
Poor digestion,
nutrient malabsorption,
decreased circulation,
immune fatigue

Detoxification Impaired
Cells fatigued, repair and
rebuilding capacity reduced

Further Organ Impairment
Systemic innate intelligence impaired

Degeneration
Inability to repair and rebuild

Organ/System Dysfunction
Subtle or dramatic indications

Disease and Death
Cellular, organ, system, organism breakdown

at all, but it is my fervent hope that you will be able to approach it. From time to time you will waver in your efforts, guaranteed, but if you follow a good nutritional plan, coupled with a regular exercise regimen and a more active lifestyle, you will certainly move closer to it than you may have ever thought was possible.

It doesn't take much to instigate change in your life, but it takes energy to create energy. Once you've begun the process, you may actually start noticing a difference fairly soon, and that can give you motivation to keep putting your energy in that direction. With a little hard work and a lot of perseverance, you will start seeing real results from the changes you've made to your behavior. But before we get started on healing ourselves, let's first learn a little about how things should be working properly.

How Digestion Happens

I want to start by addressing digestion as a central issue to optimal health. It's not just because I am trained as a nutritional therapist, but because I believe that proper digestion is the cornerstone to the foundations of optimal health. When a client comes in to my clinic, they may present to me a variety of symptoms and conditions, but the first thing I want to look at is their digestive health. When we can resolve digestive issues, whether by using supplements to restore gut health or by modifying their diet to include more nutrient-dense properly-prepared foods, often their symptoms and conditions begin to magically subside on their own.

Some people consider the topic of digestion as a fairly messy process that they just don't want to know about. It's certainly not anything that is discussed in polite company, it's never mentioned around the dinner table, and it's only spoken about in hushed tones whenever others are present. That rules out just about every occasion, and so people end up not talking about it at all. There is no better time for discussion than the present, and I'll be more than happy to guide you through it. It's something I work with every day, and as a person who eats and digests food, you should know more about it as well.

When I give talks on nutrition, I often like to engage my audience by asking them what they think is the first part of the body involved in the digestive process. Some might say the stomach, others guess the mouth or teeth, but almost nobody offers up the answer I am looking for, which is the brain. When you smell food, think about food, look at a picture of food, rummage through the fridge, or open a restaurant menu, your brain has already gone on high alert, sending signals to every part of your body that you just might be getting some food soon. Sorry, false alarm. You just walked by the donut shop again. Good work, though. Keep walking.

Usually when I lecture on these early stages of digestion, I find that my mouth begins to salivate. I excuse myself as I swallow, and I notice audience members swallowing as well. That's how powerful this response is. Just talking about food can bring on a Pavlovian response in all of us. Eating is an instinctive drive that comes from the oldest part of our reptilian brain. Every animal knows how to put food into its mouth and render it into a state where it can be digested appropriately. Iguanas on the Galapagos Islands, for example, will aid their digestion by eating seaweed mixed with seawater, and then lay out on sunbaked rocks to cook the seaweed as it sits in their bellies. We all learned at an early age how to eat, but few of us know what actually happens once we have swallowed our food.

I like to think of digestion as an assembly line process (and a heckler once quipped that it's more like a disassembly line). Think of how cars are made, for example. At the front of the assembly line, workers put the chassis together, and they send it down the line to others who add the engine, the tires, the body, the interior, and so on, until a fine running automobile rolls off the end of the line. If the workers at the front of the line don't do a good job, the chassis ends up all wonky and will make the other workers down the line work harder to, say, fit the engine to the chassis, or else they simply can't do their jobs at all. Chaos ensues, and a similar chaos is happening inside your body when the process is not right.

It all starts with each bite of food that goes into your mouth and how you chew it. Consider that chewing your food is the one part of the digestion process over which you have 100% control. Once your food has been swallowed, it's up to the rest of the digestive tract to decide what to do with it. Maybe you've been told by either or both of your parents to slow down when you eat and to chew your food more slowly. Maybe they were just repeating what they were told when they were young, but there are actually some sound scientific principles behind that.

There are three main digesting enzymes, and there are others as well, but we'll keep it to just these three for the purposes of this discussion:

- protease, for digesting proteins into amino acids
- lipase, for digesting fats into fatty acids
- amylase, for digesting carbohydrates into polysaccharides

All three are necessary to break down your food, but the only place that amylase is produced in any significant quantity is in the salivary glands of the mouth. If you feel behind your jawbone just below your ear, you can feel and even massage your salivary glands to the point of stimulating salivation. Salivary amylase can break down carbohydrates within seconds, but once you've swallowed that bite of sandwich, pasta, or fruit, the carbohydrates don't stand much chance of any further breakdown. The longer your food – mostly carbohydrates – stays in your mouth, the better chance it will have of being broken down to a molecular level as it proceeds down the assembly line.

If you take the time to soften each bite of food in your mouth thoroughly before swallowing, using your teeth and tongue and palate to crush and mix your food with your saliva, just doing this one simple thing can be enough to dramatically improve your digestion. People with whom I have shared this information have come back to me later, reporting that their gassiness, bloating, and flatulence have all but ended since they started using this simple technique. There are many advantages to chewing mindfully, but the main benefit is to ensure that the food that goes into your stomach has already been broken down as much as possible before moving its way down the line.

Each bite of food that you swallow is termed a *bolus*, from the Greek word for 'clod'. As you swallow, these boluses accumulate in your stomach. The stomach is lined with a thin wall of crisscrossing muscles that gently but firmly knead the boluses along with gastric juices into a slushy mixture called chyme (pronounced *kime*). You can't feel it while it's happening, which is probably why people tend to forget about the roiling tempest that is happening inside their stomachs.

Regarding the stomach for a moment, you can think of it as primarily a big bag of hydrochloric acid in the middle of your body. On a pH scale of zero to fourteen, where zero is pure acid, fourteen is pure alkaline, and seven is neutral, stomach acid ranges from 1.5 to 3 on the pH scale. That's strong enough to eat a hole in your carpet. Your stomach uses this strong acidity not only to break down the food you just ate, but also to try to kill off any food-borne pathogens that may have hitched a ride on your food. If you understand that we are only a century or so into anything resembling hygienic food handling and sanitation procedures, you won't consider this too odd.

pH scale

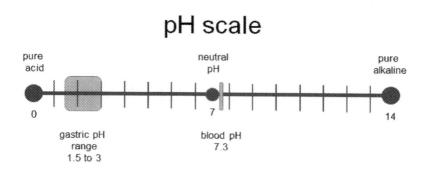

pure acid   neutral pH   pure alkaline

0   7   14

gastric pH range 1.5 to 3   blood pH 7.3

You might have experienced the wonders of chyme if you've ever had occasion to vomit. It burns your throat terribly, and that's because your throat and mouth are not prepared to handle anything so acidic. When people experience heartburn, indigestion or acid reflux, they've been told to reach for medications that will neutralize the acidity of their stomach in an effort to "put out the fire." This approach could not be more wrong. A typical cause for problems of this sort is called *hypochlorhydria*, a condition, usually temporary, where the pH of the stomach acid is too high, and therefore not acidic enough. Instead of buffering the pH of your stomach contents with over-the-counter medications, thus defeating the purpose of gastric production of hydrochloric acid, you need to take it in the other direction. There are actually pill forms of hydrochloric acid that you can take before meals to augment and stimulate the production of hydrochloric acid in your stomach. Increasing the acidity of your stomach contents enables it to work more efficiently and is much more effective than reducing its acidity.

Another easy way to stimulate hydrochloric acid production is a small glass of water with a tablespoon of either lemon juice or apple cider vinegar, taken just before a meal. This is easy enough to incorporate into your dining ritual at home, but even when you go out to a restaurant, it's not that difficult to do either. When you are first seated and the waiter hands around menus, they are likely to ask you if there's anything you'd care to drink (preferably from the bar). It's not at all fussy to ask for just a small glass of water with a lemon wedge and no ice. Any restaurant should be able to accommodate this, and you can deftly spritz the lemon into the water as you continue to peruse the menu and enjoy sparkling conversation with your friends or family.

What Next?

Let's make our way down the assembly line. Once the stomach has broken down its contents, typically in about two to four hours, it begins to pass the contents bit by bit into the next stage, called the duodenum. This is a sort of small holding tank before the chyme can move into the rest of the small intestine, and there it is treated with a variety of chemicals. Beginning with a shot of good old sodium bicarbonate, the acidic stomach contents are buffered to a pH of around 7.3, just a shade more alkaline than neutral, enabling its safe passage through the rest of the alimentary canal. The pancreas also adds various digestive enzymes that begin the further chemical breakdown of your food into their nutritive components. The duodenum releases two important hormones, secretin and cholecystokinin (or CCK), that stimulate the liver and gall bladder to produce bile, which in turn helps emulsify fats. Bile also stimulates the intestines to induce peristalsis, the rhythmic movement of the intestinal muscles that propel their contents down the assembly line. Bile is a good thing.

Once the chyme has been properly treated, it moves into the small intestine, whose job is to extract nutrients from the stomach contents as they pass through. Most of your abdominal cavity, from the bottom of your ribs to the area between the points of your pelvis, is filled with your small intestine. The lining of the small intestine is thinner than the skin covering your eyelids, and it is lined on the inside with finger-like cells called *villi* (Latin for "fingers"). These increase the surface area of the intestinal lining and are like a vacuum cleaner sucking up molecular nutrients from what was once your dinner, and then passing them into the blood stream to be parceled out to various parts of the body.

Your autoimmune system has its headquarters in your small intestine. Your intestines, in fact, are host to colonies of enteric biota (we just call them "gut bugs") that perform much of the heavy lifting involved in the absorption and conversion of nutrients, and their subsequent transfer through your system. They are instrumental in gleaning energy from undigested carbohydrates and short-chain fatty acids. There are over one hundred trillion microbial cells in the gut, which is more than ten times the number of human cells that make up your body. Pondering the fact that we can be seen as just a walking host container for teeming bacterial colonies that are collectively greater than ourselves, and that we are only composed of about ten percent human cells, really puts our existence into a new perspective, doesn't it?

After it has completed its journey of more than twenty feet through your lower abdomen, what remains of the items you ate are by now mostly indigestible. This includes soluble and insoluble fiber as well as any remaining chunks of food that weren't properly chewed at the beginning of the assembly line. The large intestine will continue to try and extract nutrients from this, but its main purpose is to draw wastes from various parts of the body in preparation for the elimination process.

Your body is dotted with over six hundred lymph glands, and many of them lie along the outside of the large intestine. Unlike the cardiovascular system, the lymphatic system is not a closed system and does not have a central pump like the heart. It relies on the efforts of the spleen, tonsils, and thymus gland to regulate its function, but, compared to the circulatory system, lymph moves through the body very slowly. It's more of a filtration system, cleansing the blood and moving waste into the large intestine for excretion. Proper care and attention to your lymph glands is crucial to maintaining optimal health, and regular vigorous exercise is one of the best ways to provide lymphatic support.

Once the waste products – cast-off tissue cells, environmental toxins, or the detritus of yesterday's three square meals – are gathered up from various parts of the body, they move through the ascending, transverse, and descending colon for a final shot at extracting any remaining nutrients while amassing all of the body's waste products in preparation for elimination. From here, we are all quite familiar with the final stages of elimination.

Elimination

At first I wanted to avoid this part, but it bears discussion here. Growing up in a household of five boys, we never grew tired of peepee-poopoo jokes, and farting and belching were much-heralded celebratory contests. As I grew older and more genteel, the topic was to be avoided and going to the bathroom was only hinted about, at best. Now that I am in the business of healing others, I could talk about stool and urine all day.

It's important to pay close attention to what your body is excreting, because this gives us important insight into how our bodies are processing nutrients. Whenever you go to the toilet, make it a habit of looking back into the bowl to see what you have eliminated. Ever heard of the Bristol scale? It was developed by Dr. Ken Heaton of the University of Bristol as a medical aid to classify human feces into seven categories. The scale has to do with stool firmness and is a clear indicator of gut health. For example, a 1 on the scale would be hard rock-like stools that are painful and difficult to pass and usually indicate severe constipation. Occasional stools that are a 2 and 3 are common signs of brief periods of dehydration, where 4 and 5 are considered optimal. Once we get to the 6 and 7 area, the stool is almost completely liquid and we are probably experiencing a condition of bowel distress resulting in diarrhea.

When I was recovering from my period of illness, I created a simple chart that I posted on the wall in my bathroom at home. It had columns for me to enter the date, my weight, and Bristol number and color. Every day I would weigh myself after my morning movement, and I recorded the results to help track how my body was recovering. If I reported a two or three, I could easily think back and realize that I hadn't drunk enough water the day before. If it was more of a six or seven, it might have been diet-related, and I would think back on what I'd eaten recently. In either case, I would check it against the adjacent days to see if a trend was forming or if it was just a brief anomaly.

Hard stools obviously indicate constipation and loose stool indicates diarrhea, but there are other things you can learn from your stool. Does it float or sink? Floating stools often accompany gassiness and bloating with meals, which indicate improper digestion of carbohydrates that ferment in the intestines. Are they light-colored, grayish or chalky? This can be a lack of proper bile production which indicates liver distress (though it can also mean you're overusing antacids). Black, tarry stools usually reveal a serious condition of bleeding in the intestinal tract and should be seen to immediately. And if it has a consistently strong odor, you most likely have an issue with malabsorption of nutrients. If your body is unable to extract all the nutrients from the food you're eating, this can be an early indicator of things like Celiac disease, Crohn's disease, or chronic pancreatitis. Thin, ribbon-like stool can signal a bowel obstruction, anything from acute constipation to polyps or even tumors. All of these are signs that you should report this to your health care practitioner sooner rather than later.

Healthy stool has a medium brown color which mostly comes from dead tissue cells sloughed off from within the body. It is ideally smooth and soft, comes out mostly in a single piece, and a perfect specimen would be an inch or two in diameter and about eighteen inches long. It should depart your body gently and with little effort as it glides softly under the water. It will likely smell, but not too strongly. Certain foods, such as beets or spinach, can discolor the stool temporarily, and if you'd like you can reminisce on the great meal that contained these things.

Transit time is an important factor to consider. It's a measure of the time it takes for the food you've eaten to leave your body in the form of waste, and the average is anywhere between 12 to 50 hours with wide variation between individuals. Undigested food reveals a short transit time[1], and that can be an early indicator for things like chronic diarrhea, colitis, and some types of irritable bowel syndrome (IBS). It's your body's way of telling you that it can't digest your food well enough. Think of stool as your body's "CHECK ENGINE" light.

If your stool contains undigested matter, we should start by looking at the beginning of the assembly line. The first culprit might be that it wasn't properly chewed in the first place, and we can refer back to the previous section on chewing food properly. But it can also tell you something about having poor nutrient absorption, and this is something you will want to know more about by talking with your healthcare provider. Long transit times indicate a wider variety of possible conditions, from simple constipation (simple - yeah, right?) to more serious conditions such as bowel obstructions and tumors. In any case, it is something you want to discuss with a trained professional.

Constipation is a serious matter, and it's more than just not being able to poop. I had one client who'd admitted to having chronic constipation to the point that she had sometimes gone up to 21 days without a bowel movement. This is beyond just an uncomfortable obstruction. It's actually interrupting the body's natural detoxification process, and at the same time it's retoxifying you and making you sicker. Some of the best remedies for temporary constipation are proper hydration, bile salts or liver-tonifying foods such as beets to help stimulate peristalsis, along with a diet slightly higher in insoluble fiber. There are many

---

[1]   There are some foods, notably corn, with large amounts of non-digestible cellulose that can show up in your stool as a perfectly normal occurrence. There are exceptions to every stool.

over-the-counter remedies that can simply add bulk to the stool, but I would recommend against them unless you are sure all of the ingredients are whole and natural and not rife with additives and preservatives and sugars that don't make you any healthier. None of these products are any substitute for a nutrient-dense diet of properly-prepared whole foods.

Urine is another yardstick of overall health, and this is something you should notice every time you have a pee. The color of one's urine can not only give you a snapshot as to your level of hydration, it can also reveal things like an otherwise undetected disease or condition, the result of medications or supplements, or just what foods you have recently consumed. We all know of asparagus' infamous ability to make our urine have a strong smell, and how beets give urine a temporarily pinkish hue. Supplemental B vitamins can cause urine to turn a bright lemon-yellow color, regardless of your level of hydration, and some prescription medications can turn the urine various shades of blue or green or orange.

When you find yourself to be dehydrated, one well-known indicator is dark yellow urine. When you notice this, it's never a good idea to start drinking large amounts of water quickly in an effort to "catch up." This can cause the water you drank to just wash through your body before it has time to fully absorb into your system, and that will show up as clear urine within a short while. Few excreted materials are carried with it, and no matter how much water you've just chugged, you will remain slightly dehydrated until your hydration levels return to normal. There will be more in this topic later in the book.

How You Got Sick

Generally speaking, we Americans tend to be fat and sick. We have become a culture of malnourished obesity and, for the most part, we're fine with that. We consume more and our bodies utilize less. Our bellies are full, and the rest of our bodies are riddled with preventable diseases. We sit and wonder how we got here. We even tend to celebrate our predilection with junk food. When bakeries owned by Hostess Brands were shut down in 2012 by striking bakery workers who learned that their pensions had allegedly been looted by upper management, there was a greater hue and cry about the possible demise of Twinkies, Ding-Dongs, and Wonder Bread than about the whereabouts of the bakery workers' retirement fund.

We are assaulted by the shrill voice of advertising from every direction - TV, the Internet, radio, billboards, buses and cabs, mobile apps, and just about everywhere you turn. If you could put on thick eye blinders, seal your ears with wax, and bury your head under every bed pillow in the house, the sheer pressure of all the energy being directed at you to consume unhealthy food would seep through to the core of your being and compel you to march zombie-like to the nearest store for a bag of chocolatey-dipped cheesey puffs[2].

---

[2]   I take only mild *schadenfreude* in mentioning that, as of this writing, quarterly earnings for companies like McDonalds, Campbell's, and Monsanto are sharply declining. Junk food is losing its relevance, and organic produce is currently the fastest-growing supermarket section.

One message that you'll seldom hear through all this cacophony is that you have choices. The other messages are so strong that they forget to mention that you can slake your thirst with pure water better than you can with ice-cold sugary sodas or artificial sports drinks. You can snack all day long, and I often recommend it, but instead of candy or chips you can choose to snack on fruit or nuts that will restore the fiber and minerals that get lost during the course of an average day.

Modern humans seem to be the only organisms bent on their own willful destruction throughout the course of their entire lives. Annual plants, for example, will wither and die as they reach the end of their reproductive cycle. But human beings engage in behaviors that can only be described as self-destructive, and it starts from the beginning. These are behaviors that we have learned, either by following the actions of others, or through arriving at our own conclusions. Sometimes we just don't care, and we'll opt for sedentary lifestyles frosted with unhealthy food choices because we've adopted them as a more comfortable way of going through life. As a result, by some estimates[3], up to 95% of all preventable diseases are based on unhealthy lifestyle choices.

There is a Catalan proverb: "From the bitterness of disease we learn the sweetness of health." Most of us don't think much about our health until we fall ill. We go on about our lives, doing as we want, eating whatever we want, and not thinking much about all the processes going on inside our bodies that keep us alive and healthy. We feel as though we shouldn't ever have to think about being sick, that we're all ten feet tall and bulletproof. That is, until something starts to break down. We imagine everything is doing

---

I only hope that those companies will learn to retool their business models to meet consumer demand for better-quality food.

[3] US Centers for Disease Control and Prevention, "Chronic Diseases: The Leading Causes of Death and Disability in the United States" 2014

fine, and then suddenly it happens - a pain, a patch on our skin, a weakness that wasn't there yesterday. We hope that it will just go away. We don't want to imagine that it could be something serious. After all, just yesterday we were fine, weren't we? Maybe we'll just get used to it.

It's been said that Americans have the worst diet of any developed nation in the world, and that the Standard American Diet (SAD) is a recipe for chronic intestinal disease, diabetes, obesity, inflammation, sluggishness, and a wide variety of other ailments. These are not statements made lightly or without careful consideration. Although we enjoy a wealth of natural resources - broad fertile plains, abundant oceans and rivers, ample pastureland - too much of the food that is produced in this country is grown in a fairly sterile environment. Even though it's technically outdoors and subject to the whims of Mother Nature, rural family farms have given way to massive monocultural oligopolies in which only one type of product - Yellow Dent corn or Iceberg lettuce or Russet Burbank potatoes, for example - is grown on agricultural stations several thousands of acres in size and bereft of any biological diversity. When the fences around the fields carry skull-and-crossbones warning signs and the field workers have to wear respirators and hazmat suits, there's something inherently wrong in our food production methods.

Humans figured out the practice of crop rotation over eight thousand years ago, but money and technology have driven farmers to abandon this practice, opting instead for pesticides and synthetic fertilizers in an attempt to control Nature. Most of these factory farms follow a tried-and-true formula called N-P-K, which uses fertilizers that enrich the soil with nitrogen, phosphorus and potassium, while ignoring all of the other essential trace minerals that once came from producing food in a more natural environment.

Much has been written about the sorry state of our country's agribusiness. I'd like you to take the time to learn more about this on your own to find out where the food in your part of the country comes from. It's in knowing how and where our food is produced that has brought about a growing movement of self-educated consumers who have chosen to buy their food only from trusted local sources that use sustainable agricultural methods. As a result, organic produce is currently the fastest-growing supermarket section. I support this trend, and I do most of my grocery shopping at my local farmers market. Beyond the benefits to my health and to the local environment, I get the warm fuzzies from handing my money over to the people who raised and produced the food I'm going to eat.

So much of the food we eat has become so nutritionally worthless that it just serves as a placeholder in our digestive system. As we learned in a previous chapter – that food is swallowed, mushed up into chyme by the stomach, passed through the small intestine for nutrient absorption, and moved by peristalsis to the large intestine for waste removal - this process is now just passing the contents through our system to stave off an increasing hunger response, leaving little in the way of nutrients that actually get to our various organs to maintain proper function.

This is why, if you want to improve your health, you need to pay very close attention to where your food comes from and how it is made and grown. It would be better that you prepare most of your meals at home, because then you will have the greatest control over the preparation and ingredients. If you can't always do that, though, it would please me greatly to turn you into the person who blocks the supermarket aisles, peering through your reading glasses to read each and every one of the ingredients in each and every product you are planning to buy. The next step beyond this is to read all the ingredients, and then put the product back on the shelf and choose not to buy it because you don't like what you just read. Consumerism is one of the purest forms of democracy, and each purchase you make is a vote in favor of that company making more of that product. Not buying something is a vote asking them to stop making that product. We consumers forget that we hold all the cards regarding what the food producers do and don't make.

Why Most Of Us Are Unhealthy

A recent article in USA Today by Kevin Speight listed "The Top Seven Health Issues in America." These were selected using a single criterion, namely those conditions resulting in the medications most frequently prescribed to Americans.

1. Hypothyroid function
2. High cholesterol and triglyceride levels
3. Heartburn and esophageal reflux
4. Breathing disorders such as asthma and chronic obstructive pulmonary disorders
5. High blood pressure
6. Diabetes
7. Depression and anxiety

All of these are lifestyle diseases, those that we bring upon ourselves through our lifestyle choices, mostly poor diets, exposure to toxins, smoking, and lack of exercise. We are paying closer attention to advertising jingles and manufactured scents and flavors and paying less attention to what our bodies are telling us. The fact that the above list is based on the frequency of prescribed medications suggests several things:

- The patients who are receiving these medications likely went for a long time suffering with their symptoms before going to see a doctor who eventually prescribed the meds.

- Many patients might present with one or more of these conditions simultaneously, underscoring the likelihood that they have subjected themselves to years of neglect.
- Little attempt was made by medical staff to alter or even address these patients' lifestyle choices in an effort to control their symptoms.
- Physicians tend to make use of prescription medications as the primary treatment protocol for managing patients who present with these conditions.

As more and more patients turn up in hospitals across the country with such a broad variety of complaints, healthcare workers end up overwhelmed by their caseloads and turn to the path of least resistance regarding patient management. This often comes in the form of a tried-and-true pill that makes the symptoms of the disease go away while creating a whole new set of problems that the patient did not have prior to seeking treatment. I could get on a soapbox about how there is more money to be made in "researching" diseases than in actually curing them, but perhaps I'll leave that for another book and take this time to maintain my focus on how just changing one's diet, even slightly, can bring about great changes in one's overall well-being.

I've mentioned that if you are eating the Standard American Diet, you are on a diet that is unhealthy. This is because much of the food sold and consumed here is heavily processed and is adulterated with so many things that our bodies were never meant to digest. Most of the added chemicals are there just to extend the shelf life of the product, increasing the time that it can sit in a silo, a warehouse, or on store shelves before making its way to your dinner table. Think about this for a minute: if you were to make the same dish from scratch that you could buy in of a box or can, would you add any of the preservatives or artificial colorings or flavorings that you see in the fine print on the label of that prepared food? You probably wouldn't even know where to obtain them, and many of them are not sold to the public anyway.

I'm originally from the South, so let me use a common staple down there to illustrate a point. It's one of my guilty pleasure foods, and when done right it is a truly amazing dish: Southern Fried Chicken. If you've ever tried making this at home, it's a huge hassle. First you have to procure, slaughter, pluck and cut apart a chicken, and then do something with the entrails and feathers. Next, you'll need a very large amount of oil and a pot or skillet large enough to fry it all in. You have to bread the chicken parts with flour and seasonings, fry the pieces in very hot oil that can be dangerous for an inexperienced cook, and then drain them on several layers of paper towels before finally sitting down to eat. After dinner, you have a pretty good mess in your kitchen, with droplets of oil spattered all over the range, dusty flour on your countertops and floor, a greasy smell throughout the house and a large amount of hot dirty oil to deal with. Or you can just order it by the bucket at a drive-up window, easy-breezy.

The fact that we have distanced ourselves so far from the cooking process and made labor-intensive home-cooked foods like fried chicken become a regular fast-food staple of our diet is one of the culprits here. For so many people, cooking is seen as a chore that is as odious as it is painstaking, and with so many restaurant choices readily available to us, there seems to be no reason to even bother with cooking. As of this writing, restaurant revenues have finally outpaced supermarket revenues, suggesting that people are going out to eat more often than they are preparing food in their home. As a result, many people now feel that they would rather take a gamble on their health than to ever attempt to cook at home.

Dining out every now and then is fine, and I look forward to the mountain of mail from restaurateurs that I will surely get over this, but in my opinion we've been given so many options that a lot of us decide to take the easy path to filling our hungry tummies.

It makes me think of people who move to the country and have wild animals living near them. They feed the deer, raccoons, and even bears that pass by as though they were family pets, to the point where the animals become increasingly dependent on humans for their food and eventually lose their ability to hunt for food in the traditional way. We, too, have lost our ability to take charge of our own nutritional needs and are accustomed to others handing us treats.

All of this change is only a couple of generations old. It's relatively new in the course of human history. Your parents and grandparents may have resorted to using foods of convenience, but in the generations before that, preparing meals was something that could approach being a full-time job. There was once a working class, a part of which had to slave away all day over a hot stove to prepare and serve meals for their betters. Later, food preparation in most families had Mom in the kitchen, cranking out three meals a day along with snacks and desserts. This situation hardly exists any more, and with so many convenient options for other people to cheaply make your food for you, why should it? When you think about it, we all now have the equivalent of cooks and servants and butlers and maids who will do all the food preparation, cooking, serving and cleaning up afterward. All we have to do is sit down and place our order, and the food comes to us in a few minutes after which we can get back to our busy day. I've worked in many restaurants during my day and even owned one for a while, and it's odd to think that they (we) have created an environment that suggests that they can cook better, serve better food, and provide you with a better dining experience than you can have in your own home. Dining out has become the norm for many people, and eating at home is turned into a drudgery. It's always confounded me that so many people these days don't even know how to cook.

How To Cook

I never intended to turn this into a diet book or a recipe book. If you never learned to cook, I urge you to seek out a few good recipes that suit your tastes, and then start learning to prepare and cook your own food. This is a great foundation for taking charge of your own health. Find a few good recipes that are tasty, that are not too complex and don't take up too much time, and these will give you a good basis for creating your own nutritional health. There is no shortage of books on the topic of what you should eat, and each one claims to have the best all-around diet that will melt away those excess pounds with little or no effort. Some even have a lot of good sound information, and so I urge you to look through the titles and skim the content to find one that most clearly speaks to you, and go with what works.

One good way to learn how to cook is to just start cooking things. Find things you like, try a few new recipes every now and then, get out a sharp knife and a hot pan and see what goes well together. You might end up throwing away some truly inedible concoctions, but you could also just as easily find something you enjoy making and that tastes great to you. Preparing and cooking food is a richly sensuous task, and, as food author Anthony Bourdain vividly noted, cooking a meal is one of the most intimate things you can do for someone else, second only to oral sex.

Another recommendation I have is that you use a recipe as a launching point, and then modify it to suit your tastes. You may end up with a spectacular disaster that ends up in late-night pizza delivery, but that's just part of the learning process. Once you've mastered a few basic recipes, you can take them to the next level and make a new signature dish that you'll come back to again and again.

Here's a loose recipe that I will share, intentionally using only broad generalities and which I urge you to take as far as you'd like to go. The measurements and ingredients are deliberately approximate, and please feel free to substitute as you see fit. You're in charge here.

No Recipe Stir-Fry

- 1 cup vegetables, chopped to medium dice
- 1 piece of meat, tempeh or tofu, sliced or cubed thinly
- 2-4 tbsp. saturated fat (butter or ghee, lard, tallow, bacon fat, coconut oil, palm oil)
- ½ cup carbohydrate (cooked rice, noodles, etc.)
- Something for a sauce (tamari, fish sauce, sriracha, sesame oil, powdered arrowroot) Seasonings to taste

1. Prepare all ingredients before starting cooking. Chop all vegetables, get out any seasonings you'll want to add, cook the rice or noodles ahead of time, prepare a sauce. The French word for this is *mise en place*, which means you'll have everything ready to go before you need it.
2. Place a wok or skillet on the cooker and set the heat to its highest level.
3. Once the pan is hot, add some of the oil and the protein component. Stir this around until it is cooked thoroughly and showing some browning on the outside. Remove from pan and set aside for later use.

4. Add more oil to the pan, and then add in the vegetables. Stir them around well, and if your pan is hot enough, you should hear a delightful sizzling sound coming from the pan.
5. To hasten cooking, add a small amount of water, wine, stock or other liquid to the pan and cover for a few minutes to steam-cook.
6. Remove the lid and push the contents to the edge of the pan.
7. Add more oil to the center of the pan and add your carbohydrate component.
8. Let it sit and brown up for a moment, then stir together to combine.
9. Add the cooked protein and continue stirring.
10. Add the prepared sauce and toss well.
11. Serve piping hot.

A few notes about cooking at this level:

- Each individual serving of meat should be about the size of the palm of your hand, approximately four ounces or so.
- Poly- or monounsaturated fats (olive oil, corn oil, canola oil and so on) are not suitable for high-temperature cooking, as their fatty acid chains will quickly break down under the heat and do more harm to you than good. The best oils for frying are ghee, coconut oil or palm oil.
- Learn to become aware of where your ingredients came from. For example, I prefer arrowroot powder to cornstarch because the majority of corn grown in this country is genetically modified.
- It's best if nothing you used came from a can, package or freezer, and if it did you'll want to make sure they contain only one or two ingredients and that none of them are chemicals. Once you begin cooking with whole, real foods, it's likely you'll lose your taste for the commercial stuff.

One thing I like about this recipe is that, because of the high heat, you are actively cooking the entire time. It's not a dish that you can put on a low simmer while you watch a TV show, but it all goes together quickly once you get your rhythm. It also causes you to use all five senses - smelling and tasting, of course, listening for changes in the cooking process, touching it (with a utensil), and looking in on it to check whether it's done.

Any good hobby should stimulate you on all possible levels, and I recommend that you look on cooking as a hobby. You have to eat anyway, so taking charge of what you eat by planning, buying, preparing, cooking, and serving it yourself becomes less of a chore when you make it into an enjoyable pastime. As with any hobby, it's all about tools and materials, time and temperature, skill and effort. If you play sports, fix up hot-rods, or build ships in bottles, you know exactly what I mean, and you can apply this same philosophy to your cooking. If bowling is your hobby, you'll soon find yourself investing in the best shoes, ball, ball bag, a team shirt, and all the other accoutrements that help you do your best. Similarly, if you buy a couple of good-quality knives, cutting boards, pots and pans, and an impressive array of kitchen gadgets, you will be better equipped to explore more in your own kitchen.

You will likely have more fun, too. If you learn to turn cooking into something you enjoy, even when you're just cooking for yourself, you create more happiness for yourself. When you invite more happiness into your life, you improve the quality of your life, and even if little else changes, your health cannot help but improve. By taking charge of your own health and becoming the master of your health condition, instead of letting it become your master, you will begin to step into a greater level of self-healing.

SECTION II

Healing

Practice then from the start to say to every harsh impression,
"You are an impression, and not at all the thing you appear
to be." Then examine it and test it by these rules you have,
and firstly, and chiefly, by this: whether the impression has
to do with the things that are up to us, or those that are not;
and if it has to do with the things that are not up to us, be
ready to reply, "It is nothing to me."

Epictetus

To move from a place of illness to wellness, you first need to prepare your self to become open to making significant changes in your life. It's not just a simple matter of substituting one type of food for another; it's a willingness to create and accept a high level of change in your own life. That does not come without a certain cost, and that cost usually comes in the form of looking deeply into your own soul and uncovering who you really are. Maybe that seems like an absurd proposition, because who can know you better than you can? You are with your self every day, living on the inside and looking back out through your own eyes into the world. The problem is that you've been on the inside too long. How much of what you see is filtered by your own thoughts and feelings, your emotions and preconceptions, your memories of the past and your acquired ability to predict the future based on what you "know" that is a result of what you have experienced from your past. It's only through casting all that aside and seeing your self for who you really are that you can begin to create true transformation and change in your life.

You will likely uncover things you'd rather not uncover, things you'd hidden away and hoped never to see again. Perhaps it was in the way you reacted to a difficult situation. Did you run away and hide from it, did you react with anger and violence, did you laugh it off and act as though it never happened? All of these responses might seem perfectly natural and reasonable in and of themselves. But are they the result of the patterns you keep repeating over and over again? Do you have the expectation that life will respond in a different way each time you react to its challenges?

The world is a mirror of your own behavior, and it reflects back to you what you are putting out to the world. If you've ever spent much time around people who are always complaining, always angry, always cracking jokes, you might start to notice that your behavior starts to match theirs. It's perfectly natural to want to be genial with others in order to not rock the boat, but when we do that, we tend to lose sight of ourselves in the process. Another thing we lose sight of is how others are behaving whenever we are around, and when we look at our behavior objectively it can reveal to us how our behavioral patterns work.

Sometimes when I would be working on something, say, repairing a table, I found that my reaction when things were not working out was to growl and curse at it. The reaction I got from other people around me was that they were horrified by my behavior, when all I was trying to do was make the screw fit into the hole without dropping it. Was I really all that bad? I didn't think so, but the situation had shown them a side of me that they'd never seen before, and they reacted to it.

Dr. Carl G. Jung, the father of modern-day psychotherapy, had this to say about change:

> *"There is no coming to consciousness without pain. People will do anything, no matter how absurd, to avoid facing their own soul. One does not become enlightened by imagining figures of light, but by making the darkness conscious."*

To get to the core of what change can look like for you, it's important to go back to the earliest time you can remember, and find a story that illustrates the types of behavior you have carried on into your current life. Here is mine: Since I was born in October, my mother actually fudged on my age to get me into the first grade earlier. She later told me that she didn't want me to wait another year, putting me a year behind my older brother and making me so much older than the other kids in my classes. So, while Mom was busy lying to the registrar, I was sat at a small child-size table with two other kids who were around my age, a boy and a girl. I remember them being dressed nicely, as was the custom in that day. On the table were the usual things to keep kids occupied, including crayons and coloring books. I excitedly grabbed a coloring book and a crayon and started having fun coloring in it, until the boy nudged the girl and told her, "Look at how he holds his crayon." The girl gave him a knowing glance.

I noticed that I had been holding my crayon in my fist, like an unschooled neonate, where they were both holding it between their fingers like a pen, as they'd been taught. I immediately made up a long list of reasons for why he would make a comment like that.

"They're all smarter than me."

"They're all ahead of me."

"I never seem to know what's going on."

"I can't trust my own judgment."

"I never do things the right way."

"I'd better just wait and see what everyone else does, and then do as they do."

It was at that point I put down my crayon and stopped coloring. I had allowed myself to be defeated by those other kids. As I grew older, I came to realize that many situations in my life ended up with me drawing the same conclusions, telling myself the same stories, and making the same judgments: that everyone else knows more than me and I can't trust myself to do things in my own way. Whenever I found myself in a new situation - and, growing up in an Army family and always being the new kid in school, that was a frequent event - I fell back into those same old stories and judgments, and in my head I repeated them to myself over and over. Each new event that reinforced those messages ingrained them more deeply into my reality; that is, what I'd made my reality to be.

Of course, those stories aren't true at all. I can have moments of exquisite brilliance, I can take great risks without failing, and I can have understandings of things in ways that others don't. Any of us can have all that and more. But through most of my life, I chose to believe the exact opposite. Most of the decisions I made in my life had been dominated by an upset five-year-old.

Once I came to that realization, I saw my previous life for what it had been. It was an invented life, not a real life. I had made up stories and drawn conclusions that weren't true, and then proceeded to live out my life according to the dictates of all of those untruths. I had chosen to live my life based on information that was completely faulty, and, even worse, for many years I had lived in the "reality" that that's just how life is for me. I felt that I was powerless over my fate.

Parts of the story are true. I really did hold my crayon in my fist, and the boy really did say that. At least, that's how I remember the story, and I'm sure that if you were able to locate the boy and girl now, more than fifty years later, and ask them about this little episode, they would have no recollection of it at all. Our interaction had no effect on them whatsoever, but it changed my entire view of the world for the nearly five decades that followed.

Perhaps you have a similar event from your past. Perhaps there was something that had upset you early on and caused you to create false information and draw faulty conclusions around it, and you have lived your life thus far based on that information and those conclusions. Certainly, the events from your life are not going to be the same as mine, and the stories you made up around it are going to have different details and different outcomes.

Try thinking back to when you were young, the youngest age you can remember, when you had an event that changed your whole way of thinking. Maybe you were denied something you thought you should have, or maybe someone you liked treated you poorly, or maybe you broke something accidentally and caught hell for it. Later in life, perhaps something similar happened which caused the same reaction in you, reinforcing the same untrue stories about your self and making them all the more real to you. As life keeps happening to you, you apply that same template - whatever it may be, in your case - to reassure your self that your false stories are somehow still holding true.

Each of us has at least one story like this. It controls us and restricts us from reaching our greatest potential. It's what keeps us within a victim consciousness and prevents us from becoming the masters of our own lives. These stories have become so ingrained in our every thought and action that we don't even realize that they exist anymore. They have become so real to us that there seems to be no alternative, and we settle into a life of resignation and cynicism. We can't change who we are, can we?

Enjoying optimal health is a by-product of casting off the negative stories from our past that we've carried around with us all these years, and it starts by identifying them for what they are. It doesn't come without a lot of deep soul-searching and perhaps even professional help, but it won't happen if you don't start and if you don't give it your all. A willingness to be brutally honest with your self is what's required here, with a sincere heart, an open mind, and a pure life energy that is dedicated to returning to who you truly are.

Once you awaken to the fact that you carry all these harmful stories inside you that are keeping you from your best health, you no longer have any reason for them to occupy space within you. You have drawn back the curtain and revealed them for what they are, and it's not been impressive. You have taken away their power to control you any further.

It's time to evict those harmful stories and create a clearing in the space they once occupied. Imagine that the space that they once occupied in your mind is now just blank, empty space. Close your eyes and think of that empty space as being like a freshly-cleaned floor, with nothing on it; no furniture, no rugs, no dust or grimy build-up. All of that has been cleared away and the space is completely empty, like a blank canvas. Now imagine what kinds of things you can put into that space, which is basically anything and everything that you desire. You can put anything you've ever wanted to be or do or have into that clearing, and the stories are no longer there to make those new things impossible.

There's an important distinction to be gleaned from within that last sentence. Being, doing and having are the proper order in which to approach this, but most of us tend to get it backwards. We believe if you **HAVE** all the things in life that you would like, you will be able to **DO** whatever you want, and then you will get to **BE** who you aspire to be. That's completely the opposite of how it works. If what you want, for example, is to be debt-free, or to have a better relationship with your family, or to lose thirty pounds, if you change your way of thinking you will start **BEING** a person who **IS** those things. By **BEING** within the mindset of someone who **IS** debt-free, you will change your thinking to someone who does not accrue additional debt. By **BEING** someone who has better relationships, you start by **BEING** someone that others can trust and rely on. By **BEING** someone who can lose thirty pounds, you make changes to your lifestyle habits that will help losing all that weight become more realistic. By thinking in the mindset of **BEING** that person, you will start **DOING** the things that sort of person does. Before long, as your behavior changes you will start **HAVING** the things that type person has. **HAVING** the things you want in life might be the ultimate goal, but it's not the first step along the path. You need to start out by behaving as a human **BEING**, without focusing on being a human **DOING** or a human **HAVING**.

Now is a good time for you to do a little exercise. Take out pen and paper and write down three things that you would like to **BE**. If you think of more than three things, write them down, too, but make sure they are not things you want to **DO** or **HAVE**. You may want to **HAVE** a new car or **DO** more adventurous things, but if those are your goals, what would you need to **BE** in order to **DO** or **HAVE** those? Go ahead and write those down, because they will become something you can review and refer back to later. You can check against your actual behavior to see if you are **BEING** who you want to **BE,** and whether that new way of **BEING** is moving you more into new ways of **DOING**. The **HAVING** comes later.

This whole process becomes an exercise in developing and strengthening your will. There is a famous psychological study that was conducted at Stanford University called the Marshmallow Test, which speaks to the human nature of self-control. Young children were brought into a room and sat at a table that held a plate with just one marshmallow. The kids were told that they would be left alone for a few minutes, and during that time they could either eat the marshmallow or leave it alone. If they didn't eat the marshmallow, when the proctor returned they would get a second marshmallow and could eat them both without consequence. If they ended up eating the first marshmallow, however, they would not get a second one. The researchers found that the children who were able to wait for the second marshmallow tended to grow up having better life outcomes, as measured by such diverse things as educational attainment, SAT scores, body mass index, and other standards.

Whether or not the test subjects ate the marshmallow makes no difference in determining their destiny, and the good news is that self-control can be a learned behavior. Grown-ups can use it to tackle the burning issues of modern middle-class life, such as learning to go to bed earlier, to control their anger better, to not check their phones obsessively, or to cut down on sweets.

Part of what adults need to learn about self-control can be seen in the videos of these young test subjects. The children who went on to succeed are the ones who managed to turn away from the marshmallow, push it away, or pretend it's something inedible like a piece of rubber instead of just sitting there staring down the marshmallow. They mentally transformed that marshmallow into something with less of an attraction to them. Adults can use similar methods of distraction and distancing. For example, don't stare at that breadbasket all through dinner; just remove it from the table. In moments of emotional distress, try imagining that you're viewing your self from outside, or consider what someone you admire would do in your place. When someone offers you a slice of chocolate cake, look upon it as if it has just been colonized by worms.

There are two opposing parts of the brain: a hot part demanding immediate gratification (the limbic system), and a cooler, more goal-oriented part (the prefrontal cortex). The secret of self-control is to train the prefrontal cortex to kick in first. To do this, use specific if-then plans, like "If it's before I have to be at work, I won't check my email" or "If I feel like having something sweet, I will drink a glass of water instead." When you do this repeatedly, this buys you a few seconds to at least weigh your options.

The point isn't to be robotic and never eat sweets again; it's to teach your self how to summon up self-control whenever you want it, and to be able to make those actions turn into long-term habits. Please be aware that self-control alone doesn't guarantee success. People also need a burning desire – a goal that gives them a reason to activate these skills. College students may all have the determination in the world to get into graduate school, but the best ones also have a deeper question that they want to answer in their work, which may sometimes be something that has come from their own lives.

We often do outrageous, flamboyant, conspicuous things and then say later that we were "embarrassed" by what we did We confuse the word "embarrassment" with feelings of shame over what we may have done, but another way to look at feelings of embarrassment is to say that we have *surpassed* our selves. For just a moment, we went beyond the boundaries of our egos and then, suddenly, looked around and saw that we are standing at the edge of the stage, with a bright spotlight shining only on us, and with ten thousand people watching. We might want to quickly retreat back into our safety zone, apologizing profusely for acting the way we did. I say 'we' because I have to include myself in that group – I am as imperfect as anyone else. But practicing the act of surpassing your self and your ego will inspire you to shed the bonds of your past and enable you to move into something new.

It takes a great deal of fortitude and determination to find the motivation to elicit change in your life. Sadly, this is often precipitated by a near-catastrophic illness or condition that serves as a wake-up call - if you're lucky. I had a similar wake-up call, and I would not wish that level of illness on anyone. If you think your health just might be slipping a little, it is. If you think that your old ways of going through life aren't serving you very well any more, they aren't. If you think you might need some help, you do. The sooner you act on it, the easier it will be. The patients mentioned at the beginning of this section, for whom all those medications were prescribed, waited too long.

It's okay to ask for help. We so seldom do this, and I find this most common in the male population. It's a common stereotype that men, in general, will act as though everything's OK and that they've got everything under control. In his book **Under Saturn's Shadow: The Wounding and Healing of Men**, author James Hollis tells us, "Men collude in a conspiracy of silence whose aim is to suppress their emotional truth." Throughout our lives we hear messages coming from all around us, harmful messages that manipulate our thoughts and actions to conform to whatever advertisers tell us are good or healthy or fun or that represent appropriate behavior.

Men live through a litany of harmful messages throughout their lives, and their subtext runs along the lines of this:

"You have to be strong!"

"You're not hurt that bad!"

"Get back to work!"

"Don't be such a wimp!"

"Don't let them see you crying!"

Women get harmful messages throughout their lives as well, but they are more like this:

"You're not pretty enough!"

"You're not thin enough!"

"You're not fashionable enough!"

"You're not happy enough!"

"You're not enough!"

One approach to these messages is to simply acknowledge and observe them without reacting. You don't need to act on them now, just step back and take a look at them. You can acknowledge them, hold them up like slips of paper to pin to your wall, and stand back and take a good look at them. "Mm-hmm, yep, that's what those messages are saying, all right," you can think to yourself as you observe without judgement. But consider that they're just words. There's no action for you to take with them right now. Just step back and look at them objectively.

If you were to try and evaluate them for what they mean, you will probably end up in frustration. There is no truth to them. All the messages I listed above, all the stories we're told as we're growing up and that we've carried out into our adult lives and reinforced over and over again as the same things keep happening to us again and again, are just stories. They're made up. They're not even true stories. So what would happen if you cleared away all of those false stories and just ignored them? You may think that you can't just shut off the many voices in your head that keep reinforcing those stories every waking hour of the day, but what if you could, even just for a moment? I believe that you would find a clearing in all that undergrowth, among all the harmful lies that we've accepted as truth. In that clearing, you are able to create anything and everything that you want. Go into that clearing now and shout it out as loudly as you can!

"I am awesome!"

"I am enough!"

"I am perfect just the way I am!"

"I have unlimited power and ability!"

"No one can stop me from doing anything I want!"

As you build something new for your self inside that clearing, the clearing becomes larger and larger. Repeat your affirmations enough times and they begin to displace the negative stories and push them out of the way to make room for your new stories. The more you do this, the more your body and brain will respond positively.

Maybe this isn't the best analogy I can provide, but as you can tell by now I work well within the framework of analogies. Adolf Hitler wrote this in **Mein Kampf**:

> *"The most brilliant propagandist technique will yield no success unless one fundamental principle is borne in mind constantly and with unflagging attention. It must confine itself to a few points and repeat them over and over. Here, as so often in this world, persistence is the first and most important requirement for success."*

You won't often find me quoting freely from **Mein Kampf** [4], but this statement certainly bears closer examination. We repeat lies over and over again, and when things happen that don't go our way we recycle those lies as a way of reinforcing them. "See, I told you that would happen," we scold ourselves each time we act out a familiar scenario, and we confuse hindsight with premonition. We become resigned and cynical; resigned that it's just the way things go and there's nothing we can do about it, and cynical about our abilities to create significant change in our lives. But do you want to continue repeating negative messages over and

---

[4]   I sincerely do not wish to validate any of Hitler's efforts or to let this slip into *reductio ad Hitlerium*, but here we go. I had originally planned to use a quote that is frequently attributed to Joseph Goebbels about how you can repeat a lie often enough to make it become the truth, but in my research for this book I learned that Goebbels never said anything like that. Enter Hitler, with my deepest apologies.

over in your mind, or would you prefer to repeat positive messages that can not only lift your spirits momentarily but can contain the potential for creating significant and permanent change in your life?

I don't think most people consciously know and understand which things are best for them and then consciously act to the contrary, but it happens all the time in our unconscious minds. It's in the reinforcing power of strong positive affirmations that we begin to reverse the polarity of our thoughts, which then play out in our words and our actions. If the negative thoughts get more airplay in our minds, we continue to play them out in what we do and say. You may have run across people like this who are never happy, always grumbling about something or another, always being the victim. If, instead, you can outweigh the negative voices with positive voices - "I have infinite wisdom and beauty!" "I hold limitless power!" "Making mistakes helps me to move forward!" - soon you will begin to believe them, and you will act in ways that will bear out those new beliefs.

I knew one fellow, now deceased, who told me that every morning when he woke up he looked at himself in the mirror and said, "I love you." To some people it sounds corny and precious, something you could never see your self doing. But what if you did? What if you made a personal challenge to start doing that every morning for a hundred mornings? What if you also did it every night before you went to sleep? What if you just did it? Do you think you would be a different person after a hundred days?

Beginning a program of self-love and self-acceptance is one way to begin the process of getting over your self, and by that I mean getting beyond your ego. I often hear the words of my father, whose background was in aeronautical engineering, who taught me several of the laws of physics, including the laws of inertia. One of them states that it takes more energy to start something in motion than it takes to keep it in motion. If you've ever had to push a stalled car, you know what I mean. You usually can't just push on it to get it going, but if you start out by gently rocking it you will easily start rolling along. This is the same thing I am suggesting here. You can't expect to go from a life of fast food on the sofa and step directly into a life of granola and cross-fit classes. I know, because I tried it several times and failed.

So, as a nutritional therapist, I want to "stick with the foundations," as we say, and assume that any sort of illness, malady, disorder, or condition that you are experiencing at any given time can be attributed to and resolved by what you are eating or not eating, and what you ought to be eating or ought not to be eating. We need to take it even further from there, though, because if we want to create a complete transformation in our lives, we need to look at it from other perspectives as well; not only what to eat, but how, when, where, and why to eat. This section will help equip you with more of the knowledge you will need to take the next step forward into your own transformation.

What To Eat

It's difficult for me to tell people what they should and should not eat. I do it anyway, but there is so much emotion tied up in food that my clients will run the gamut of feelings around my suggestions. We want to hold on to our strong emotional attachments to food – the fond memories of our childhood or of holiday events; being rewarded with food, especially sweets, as a child; eating specific foods at certain events or on certain holidays – such that I can't expect anything like perfect adherence to my recommendations. We might tell ourselves, "But I need something sweet after a spicy meal," or, "I always eat popcorn when I go to the movies." We accept that a cheeseburger and a Coca-Cola are the ideal pairing. There are specific food events around watching the Super Bowl, for celebrating Thanksgiving or Passover, for when you're at happy hour, and many more.

Here's the good news. The human body, as I've said, is remarkably strong and resilient. You can adhere to a good clean healthy lifestyle, then go and have something like a slice of birthday cake and not immediately die. You might feel some effects if your body is not accustomed to that amount of sugar and refined complex carbohydrates, but, barring known sensitivities and allergic conditions, for the most part you'll recover nicely.

So - what exactly should you eat and not eat in order to enjoy optimal health? The shortest answer that I can give you, for starters, is to cut out refined sugar in all forms, along with refined complex carbohydrates, processed foods, fast foods, packaged foods, hydrogenated vegetable oils and artificial sweeteners. Sounds easy, right? To some of you, it may seem utterly impossible. If you remove all of those from your diet, what's left? Only everything else. What it leaves are whole, fresh, nutrient-dense foods that are properly prepared, or, as our ancestors called it, "food." We have gotten so far away from the original source of our food that much of the edible stuff that grows out of the ground is unrecognizable to the average consumer. And we are all consumers. It becomes, then, a matter of what we choose to consume, and if you follow the plan laid out in this book, you will teach yourself how to make better food choices that will benefit you.

Most processed foods are designed to sit on a store shelf or in a warehouse almost indefinitely, and it can be shipped around the world with little effect. In his 1975 book **Eat Your Heart Out** [5], former Texas Agricultural Commissioner Jim Hightower explains to us that higher levels of food processing provide little benefit to the quality of the food we eat, but they dramatically increase profits for the food processors. If you sell a case of tomatoes, for example, you will realize a small profit; if you sell it as canned diced tomatoes, you can use parts of the less-than-perfect tomatoes and increase your profits further; and if you mash up the rest of your crop and sell it as Chunky Spaghetti Sauce with All Natural Old World Seasonings you will garner the greatest profit of all. By way of another example, farmers might experience a dramatic drop in the wholesale price of spinach, but the price of a frozen spinach soufflé will remain the same. I don't wish to demonize anyone for wanting to make a simple profit; I just raise objections to that when it comes to our health.

You may wish to approach a radical change to your diet in graduated steps. You might, for example, be looking at a pantry

---

[5] People have asked me who my greatest influences have been. This book was one of the earliest ones I can recall that has helped to shape the way I look at how food is produced and sold to us. If you can find it, buy it!

filled with many of the items mentioned above for which you've already paid good money and that you don't want to throw out just yet. That's understandable, and that's a starting place where you can begin to phase out the things that you know aren't good for you and start replacing them with the things that will provide better benefit to your health. There are some things you may want to get rid of right away, and let me say that I'd be so delighted if you tossed your margarine in the trash right now and replaced it with real butter or coconut oil, or if you started replacing processed snacks on your shopping list with nuts and fruit.

In time, you'll begin to know which things are better replacements for the things you used to consume. You'll develop a taste for healthier foods as you lose your taste for the foods you once craved. The thought of eating a sugary dessert after every meal, oily salty snacks during the day, and high-carbohydrate processed meals will soon become foreign to you. You can teach yourself how to eat better quality foods instinctively, just as you learned to make foods that you know are bad for you somehow seem tasty. It's beyond the scope of this book to prepare specific one-size-fits-all diet plans when I've already taken a stand for bioindividuality, but the things I've mentioned above are generally good ideas for most people.

I know I'm being intentionally vague here because I know that what works for one person isn't quite right for another, but it can be easy to condition yourself to change your diet. The first step, as I've mentioned, is in wanting to make that change. Maybe you've put it off until your health condition has gotten so bad that the idea of changing your diet to improve your health has suddenly become increasingly important. Maybe you've seen other people, including friends and family members, start to lose their health over time as a result of their lifestyle choices, and it's made you start thinking more about your own health. You see them from the outside and wish that there was something you could do to help them, but you're not sure exactly what to do. You may also feel that your concerns for their health will fall on deaf ears, and so you become resigned to the fate that you cannot help them.

Sometimes it's better to choose your battles wisely and lead by example. If you become the one among your friends who always turns down dessert, who always brings your own lunch to work rather than always going out, who has noticeably lost a lot of weight and gained a lot of energy, they will probably start asking you what your secret is. It's really no secret; you can tell them that you just changed everything about everything that you eat. You can tell them that not only did you change what you eat, but you've changed how, when, where and why you eat. In short, you've taught yourself how to eat all over again. You took what little you may have known about nutrition that you'd learned in your youth and carried into your adult life, and have now chucked it out the window in favor of new and healthier eating choices that you know will be better for you. That's all.

Macronutrients

I've mentioned that I am a strong believer in the concept of bioindividuality, but I know that several concepts can be applied across the board. To understand your food better and know more about the true nature of what you are eating, it's important to break them down into groups of macronutrients. There are six major classes of macronutrients:

- Proteins
- Fats
- Carbohydrates
- Vitamins
- Minerals
- Water

The first three are the most significant, in terms of our discussion here. Everything you eat is made up of proteins, fats and carbohydrates in varying ratios. A carrot has a tiny amount of protein and fat, and the rest is carbohydrates. Conversely, a strip of bacon has a great deal of fat, quite a lot of protein and a small amount of carbohydrates.

The ratio that you want to strive for is 30:30:40, meaning your diet should consist of 30% protein, 30% fats, and 40% carbohydrates. With the Standard American Diet, most of us have gotten this completely upside-down. We might get ten to fifteen percent useable protein, less than ten percent good healthy fat because we've always been told that low-fat options are somehow healthier for you, and the rest - as much as eighty percent of our diet - is carbohydrates. We've held on to the mantra of "fat makes you fat," when in fact, if we should demonize any macronutrient, carbohydrates should get the bum rap.

Carbohydrates, in the highly refined form found in most processed foods, can cause us to gain weight and suffer all of the associated lifestyle diseases that come with obesity. The best way to achieve the 30:30:40 diet is to simply cut down on carbohydrates while slightly increasing your intake of protein and healthy fats. Because the Standard American Diet is so high in carbohydrates, it would be a good start to learn how to avoid foods high in refined carbohydrates and sugars, and then round this out with adding more protein and healthy fat to your diet.

Carbohydrates provide our bodies with energy, and they act like kindling on a fire. They tend to burn up quickly and require frequent replenishment in order to keep the fire going. It explains why you can eat snacks that are high in carbohydrates and an hour later still feel like snacking again. This, coupled with a sedentary lifestyle, will keep us hungry without properly burning off the calories we're receiving from our high-carbohydrate foods. It's where constant snacking on processed foods can turn into addictive behavior, and don't think for a moment that the companies who make all those snacks don't know that. They want you to keep buying their product, regardless of their effect on your health.[6]

Fats, on the other hand, are more like logs on a fire. They burn slowly and create a longer-lasting form of energy that will sustain us through our daily activities. Followers of the Paleo Diet understand that our ancestors from thousands of years ago used fatty foods to keep their bodies going until they could capture the next mastodon to bring back to the tribe. Increasing your

---

[6] So sue me.

level of fat and protein intake, while simultaneously lowering your carbohydrate intake, can help to quell the hunger response by increasing the satiation response, and thus keeping you from snacking and overeating. You will begin to notice that you feel hungry less often, and excess weight will begin to slowly melt away. Who would have thought that bacon is something that can help you slim down?

Fat

Fat is a word I would love to destigmatize and reclaim as a useful word in anyone's vocabulary. We use euphemisms to get around talking about dietary fat, but to your body it's pretty much all the same. As I lecture on the concept of having thirty percent of your diet coming from fat, people's jaws drop as if they think that I am suggesting they begin guzzling vats of rancid fryer oil. It's a part of my lectures that gives me great personal amusement, because it's so common for us to eschew fat in all forms that the idea of increasing our intake of dietary fat has become comically repulsive.

Since the middle of the 20th century, we've all been told what I consider a whopping big lie: "fat makes you fat." What this is saying is that fat, in any form, is what makes you put on weight and thus look objectionable to others. We've been conditioned to opt for low-fat choices almost instinctively - chicken instead of beef, skim milk instead of whole milk, "Lite Options" instead of whole natural foods. The problem with removing fat from normal foods is a reduction in what food scientists call 'mouthfeel'. When your mouth's highly-refined nerve endings sense fat, they signal the hypothalamus to dial back the hunger response and increase the satiation response, causing you to eat less and, ostensibly, to lose weight or at least not gain weight so quickly.

Foods that are presented as low-fat or non-fat omit a significant component that provides long-burning calories – the fat. Your body receives dietary fat and sends a signal, through a type of hormone called leptin, to the hypothalamus in the brain to reduce the hunger response. Without this signal coming from normally-occurring dietary fat, we would find our food rather bland and uninteresting, and so they make up for the reduced mouthfeel by just adding various forms of sugar. Read the fine print on your favorite brand of yogurt and watch as the sugar count starts to add up. It may just say sugar outright, or it may call it fructose, maltose, dextrose, lactose and so on, but to your body it's all sugar.

Near where I live, there is a large supermarket whose dairy section includes a 32-foot section of nothing but yogurt. The last time I looked, I could only find two brands that offered some sort of full-fat variety; the rest were all low-fat or non-fat versions of what was once a healthy product. Some contained more sugar per ounce than a soft drink or a candy bar. Coupling that with yogurt made from pasteurized milk, processed fruit, and artificial sweeteners gives you a little plastic cupful of nutritional worthlessness.

The first type of fat you will want to cut out of your diet immediately is all forms of hydrogenated vegetable oils. As a commercial product, these start out as natural vegetable oils such as canola, palm, soybean, or corn oil that have been extracted using harsh chemical solvents. All of these solvents that are used in creating processed vegetable oils have detrimental effects on human health and have no place in the modern human diet. Non-hydrogenated oils added to foods would become rancid quickly, and this would increase the cost to the manufacturer.

When creating these oils, first they are heated anywhere from five hundred to one thousand degrees under several atmospheres of pressure. Then a catalyst, typically a metal such nickel, platinum or even aluminum is injected into the oil for several hours. As these materials bubble up into the oil, the molecular structure of the oil increases in density and rearranges its molecules so that instead of being a liquid at room temperature it becomes either solid or semi-solid. This turns the natural vegetable oils, which can quickly become rancid with exposure to oxygen or light, into either partially hydrogenated or fully hydrogenated oils – the so-called trans-fats – that will remain shelf-stable for years.

The molecules in this product are now closer to cellulose or plastic than to natural vegetable oil. In fact, hydrogenated vegetable oil is just one molecule away from plastic. When you eat anything containing this material, just as the oil is now thicker and more viscous, your blood becomes thicker and more viscous. The heart now has to work so much harder to pump this thicker blood throughout the system. This is one of the ways that consuming hydrogenated oils contributes to high blood pressure.

In some studies[7], it has been shown that such oils contribute to elevated cholesterol levels because they actually scar the internal walls of the arteries. This is primarily due to the elements such as nickel that are used in the hydrogenation process. As the product scrapes its way through your circulatory system it creates inflammation of the arterial walls. This causes your body to send cholesterol into your bloodstream to try and patch the damaged walls of the arteries, which becomes the primary cause for a build-up of arterial plaque. As the walls are continually scarred and cholesterol dutifully continues to do its job of patching the wounds, this slowly constricts the opening for blood to flow through, making your heart work even harder and placing a greater strain on your heart until the heart eventually wears out. Cholesterol takes the fall for contributing to atherosclerosis, but the real culprit is a diet high in hydrogenated vegetable oils that create vascular inflammation, and they are in nearly all processed foods.

Natural oils have their own enzymatic activity occurring in them, which is what causes them to go rancid at room temperature.

---

[7]   "The negative effects of hydrogenated trans fats and what to do about them", Kummerow, Fred A., Atherosclerosis, Volume 205, Issue 2, 458 – 465

When natural foods use their own enzymes to break themselves down in your body, they require less of your body's enzymes to do the same job. Trying to digest this plastic-like hydrogenated oil takes a huge amount of enzymes from your system, but your body never really succeeds because it's a substance that is not natural and that your body is not designed to absorb. Such foreign substances can often cause a false immune response, which places further strain on your immune system and which can promote inflammation and decrease your overall immunity.

To help avoid the vagaries of hydrogenated oils, try eating more foods that are raw or lightly cooked to keep them as close to their original natural state as possible. This means choosing more fruits and vegetables including organic local meats. It also means becoming a diligent label-reader and checking everything you buy that's packaged and processed. You especially want to make sure to avoid products with hydrogenated oils and other harmful ingredients such as high fructose corn syrup. Just because a package has the words "natural" or "organic" on the label doesn't mean that it's necessarily a healthy food. Packaged and processed foods labeled as organic might be considered "less harmful" but are not truly as healthy as they could be. To be truly healthy means that a food contains its own naturally-occurring vitamins, minerals, enzymes, and all the other nutrients that are present.

In 2013 the US Food and Drug Administration issued a notice[8] stating that " ...industrially-produced trans fatty acids, or trans-fat, are not generally recognized as safe (GRAS) for any use in food based on current scientific evidence establishing the health risks associated with the consumption of trans fat ...." So this is not just Mean Old Jeff vaguely telling you that hydrogenated vegetable oils are somehow bad for you. Even the FDA, an agency

---

[8]   "Tentative Determination Regarding Partially Hydrogenated Oils; Request for Comments and for Scientific Data and Information", Federal Register, A Notice by the Food and Drug Administration on 11/08/2013

that has dished up some questionable decisions in the past, finally concurs that trans fats, as a food additive, are not safe for you to eat.

Certain types of essential fatty acids are involved in the body's natural inflammatory and anti-inflammatory responses. The hormones called prostaglandins are a group of lipids made at sites of tissue damage or infection that are involved in dealing with injury and illness. They control processes such as inflammation, blood flow, and the formation of blood clots. They also generate sensations of inflammation, pain and fever as part of the healing process.

When a blood vessel is injured, a prostaglandin called thromboxane stimulates the formation of a blood clot to try to mitigate the damage; it also causes the muscle in the blood vessel wall to contract (causing the blood vessel to narrow) to try to prevent blood loss. There is another prostaglandin called prostacyclin which has the opposite effect to thromboxane. Prostacyclin reduces blood clotting and removes any clots which are no longer needed; it also causes the muscle in the blood vessel wall to relax, so that the vessel dilates. The opposing effects that thromboxane and prostacyclin have on the width of blood vessels can control the amount of blood flow and regulate response to injury and inflammation.

Suppose one day, heavens forfend, you happen to step off the curb wrong and twist your ankle. Your body will send an inflammatory response in the form of prostaglandins, which lead to increased circulation in the area and cause redness and swelling. Your body's next response is to quell the inflammation by sending anti-inflammatory prostaglandins. Without the appropriate balance of healthy sources of dietary fat, this is one system that you can't expect to work properly, and an improper balance of essential fatty acids is a leading cause of a lot of inflammation that shows up everywhere from joint health to atherosclerosis.

Vitamins and Minerals

We use the term "essential" - as in essential fatty acids or essential vitamins - to describe certain types of molecules that cannot be synthesized in the body and that must come from one's diet. The vitamin D family, for example, is generally not considered essential because the body can synthesize forms of vitamin D just by being out in the sunshine. Others, such as the B vitamins, must come from our diet in sufficient amounts to sustain and help carry out all of our normal bodily functions. All minerals are considered essential because the body cannot metabolize, for example, iron or calcium. Most minerals can be stored, primarily among bone tissue, but they must first have originated from the diet.

When we take vitamins and minerals, either as supplements or as part of our diet, it's not the vitamins and minerals that make us strong and healthy. Our body uses those components as building blocks to create a strong and healthy organism. It's a complicated system of checks and balances; a deficit in magnesium, for example, can disrupt the ability for calcium to properly and appropriately contract muscle tissue. The best way to keep this well-tuned machine running properly, then, is to maintain a continual intake of only the best quality of macronutrients throughout your life. It's possible to increase deficient levels of vitamins and minerals through nutritional supplements, but the best source comes from whole natural foods that are already rich in those needed macronutrients.

I know several people in the general aviation community, people who fly an airplane for fun and recreation, and none of them would think, for example, of using anything but the highest-grade fuel for their aircraft, and to always take it in for regular inspections and maintenance. Some will even opt to do the work themselves, ensuring that they are quite familiar with every nuance of every part of their aircraft. When they are flying along at an altitude of five to ten thousand feet, with the closest patch of solid ground straight below you, their lives depend on the plane's ability to fly smoothly and to land safely. Upon arrival, these same people will think nothing of loading their bodies up with fast food and soda pop, treating their own bodies with less care than they do their airplanes.

It's important that we resolve any deficiencies in vitamins and minerals sooner rather than later. In a case of advanced mineral deficiencies, it can take months or even more than a year to bring certain mineral levels back to homeostasis. Most men become deficient in zinc, for example, and women who've had children can become highly deficient in minerals and essential vitamins as their body's supply of macronutrients gets passed on to the fetus. This helps to explain why osteoporosis is so prevalent among older mothers of large families.

Water

Water is considered a macronutrient because it is vital to our survival. We can manage to live for up to two or three weeks without food, but only a couple of days without water. Chronic dehydration is perhaps the greatest nutritional deficiency facing the world today. In countries like the United States, our dehydration comes from overconsumption of diuretics like soda pop, coffee, tea, sports drinks, alcohol, and fruit juice. Water has long been my beverage of choice, even to the point of mild ridicule by my well-meaning friends when we go out to dinner, who insist that I drink something more "interesting."

The formula for knowing how much water to drink is as simple as this:

**Half your body weight in pounds =
ounces of water per day**

That's it. Step on the scale. If you weigh, for example, a hundred and twenty-eight pounds, your daily water consumption should be sixty-four ounces. If you have a favorite eight-ounce glass, drink eight of those each day; keeping a twelve-ounce glass handy will be just six a day, and so on. If you drink any of the above-mentioned diuretics, you'll need to increase your water intake by at least half the amount of diuretics you had. So, if you drank a twelve-ounce can of soda, you'll need to drink an additional six ounces of water to make up for the loss. Err on the side of more water, not less.

Some people complain that drinking all that water will cause them to go to the bathroom more frequently than they'd care to. This may be true, but only within the first few days of getting on a protocol of regular hydration. Once your body has restored its natural level of hydration, your need to excrete excess water will decrease as your organs and joints begin to store and maintain their proper hydration level. It's also better to sip your water constantly throughout the day, rather than drinking an entire glass of water in one massive gulp, which you can rightly expect to pass through you fairly quickly.

Imagine that your body is like the Mississippi River, one of the longest rivers in the world. Several large rivers – the Ohio, the Illinois, the Tennessee – branch off of it. Each of those rivers has their own complement of tributaries, and from there are smaller creeks and streams. Regular amounts of rainfall will keep them all full, but when the rains stop the creeks and streams will tend to dry up first, and the levels of the larger rivers will begin to recede. If the beds of those smaller creeks and streams go dry, they will not be able to hold their water as well when the rains return, and they will soon go dry again unless there is sufficient and constant rain to keep their streambeds saturated. Once they have had abundant and regular amounts of water, these creeks and streams can nourish the trees and plants and animals that thrive along their banks.

This is an analogy I like to use with my clients to explain how hydration helps with joint and muscle pain, especially among athletes and those of us who are getting older. Connective tissue - tendons, ligaments, cartilage - is non-vascular and is composed primarily of water and collagen. Water is the primary way in which minerals such as calcium, magnesium, zinc and sulfur can get to this tissue. In a condition of dehydration, water is not getting to the tissue and therefore cannot carry these minerals and other compounds to where it's they're needed, and waste cannot be carried out.

Water washes through your body and purifies you. It softens and protects your organs. It lubricates and helps cushion the joints, and chronic underhydration is a direct cause of chronic joint pain. In fact, an early symptom of dehydration is not a dry mouth, it's pain. For me, the onset of a light headache is my signal that I've not been drinking enough water lately. Again, in a situation like that it's not advisable to slam a full glass of water at once in an effort to make the pain go away sooner, but to slowly sip the water over a period of fifteen to twenty minutes.

You may notice when you're dehydrated that your urine is a dark yellow, and, after you've gulped down a large glass of water in an effort to "catch up," your urine runs clear. That shows you that it is passing straight through you without taking out much waste material on its way out. Slow down and drink that glass of water over a period of fifteen to twenty minutes, and let the water slowly saturate your body's creeks and streams.

Sugar

The sugar industry creates for itself a profit of over five billion dollars a year, mostly from selling a product our bodies are ill-prepared to process. Sugar contains no essential nutrients and contributes precious little to a healthy body. Added sugars like sucrose, maltose, dextrose and the infamous high fructose corn syrup add nothing but empty calories. Sugar is also the favorite food of bacteria, including the bad bacteria that can create tooth decay, inflammation, or intestinal dysbiosis.

Fructose is a particularly problematic form of sugar, particularly artificial forms of fructose such as high fructose corn syrup. Most sugars share their metabolic workload among various organs of the body – the liver, pancreas, muscle tissue – but fructose is completely metabolized in the liver. Excessive intake of artificial fructose overburdens the liver and prevents it from the many other things it needs to do. Glucose is found in every living cell on this planet, and if we do not get it from our diet, our bodies can easily produce it from other materials. Fructose, on the other hand, is different. Our bodies do not produce it and have no direct physiological need for it. We can handle fructose from natural sources like raw fruit just fine, and there is no risk of overdose from a healthy amount of fruits and vegetables. But when our livers are already overloaded with glycogen, a stored form of sugar that it derives from carbohydrates in our diet, the added fructose stresses the liver.

Fructose triggers a process in the liver called lipogenesis (from *lipo* - "fat" - and *genesis* - "creation"), which is the production of fats like triglycerides and cholesterol. Excessive intake of fructose causes an overproduction of these natural fats which results in an unappetizing condition known as "non-alcoholic fatty liver". This condition affects over 70 million Americans by causing huge spikes in insulin, our body's primary fat storage hormone. Both of these side effects of artificial fructose lead to increased metabolic disorders that drive increases in appetite, weight gain, diabetes, heart disease, cancer, dementia, and more.

Sugar also disrupts the natural production of insulin, an important hormone for blood sugar regulation. Without insulin's ability to regulate blood glucose levels, the blood becomes highly toxified by glucose which leads to some of the more serious complications from diabetes such as blindness or necrosis of the extremities. As the cells undergo a complete metabolic dysfunction, the cells become increasingly resistant to insulin's effects.

Here's an interesting story to help you understand sugar's role in modern cuisine. In Western culture, refined table sugar has only been in the diet for about four hundred years, to about the time of European colonization of the New World. At first, sugar from the colonies was ruinously expensive and highly prized by members of the upper class. Those in lower classes noticed quickly the effect that sugar had on their betters, and would actually rub coal or pitch on their teeth to imitate the rotting teeth of the people of the higher class.

It is said that it's easier to break an addiction to heroin or tobacco than it is to sugar. The addiction recovery community uses this maxim: "If you think you're not addicted to something, just try giving it up." Try eliminating refined sugar from your diet for a week and see what happens. Will you break down and indulge in a candy bar at your moment of weakness? Will you begin to notice that sugar is everywhere you turn, temptation is around every corner, and it's hopeless to get away from it? Or will you sincerely try to extract your sweet tooth and relearn how to enjoy food that is not so heavily charged with sugar?

It's a difficult process, granted, and can be one of the most difficult journeys on which you might embark, but here are the results you can expect when you quit sugar:

Reduced hunger pangs - When your body no longer relies on sugar and carbohydrates for energy, it begins to utilize longer-burning fat (which you should be increasing in your diet, as mentioned above). You find that you tend to eat less food less frequently, and you feel satiated sooner.

Headaches and fatigue are almost completely eliminated - Energy levels will stop fluctuating as your body's cycle of releasing cortisol is more naturally regulated. Without such dramatic ebbs and flows, your energy will be more constant throughout the day, instead of waking up tired, wanting to take a nap in the afternoon, and falling asleep shortly after dinner.

Fewer mood swings and a clearer mental state – By naturally regulating your blood sugar levels, you are maintaining adequate levels of the mood-regulating neurotransmitter called serotonin. Low serotonin levels can cause anxiety, insomnia, fatigue, and depression. Sugar can provide a temporary boost of serotonin, but its effects wear off quickly, resulting in the well-known "sugar high" and "sugar crash" cycles. When your body learns to naturally regulate its own serotonin levels, your emotions will become more even-keeled, much to the delight of those around you.

Rapid weight loss followed by steady weight loss -By "rapid weight loss," I mean as much as five to ten pounds within the first week followed by a steadier decrease until you begin to plateau at your optimal size and weight. An immediate cessation of processed or refined sugar intake is a near assurance of weight loss. Of course, continuing to consume natural forms of sugar from fruits and vegetables is still recommended, but once you have stopped taking in added refined sugars your body will learn to rely on burning fat for energy rather than sugar. From this you'll begin to notice a gradual but steady decline in excess body weight. For most people, about five pounds per month is a good, healthy rate at which to lose weight, and this comes about from your body's adaptation to seeking out a different energy source. It's what I did, and I lost over sixty pounds in a year.

Improved overall health - Sugar causes so much damage to nearly every organ and tissue type in our bodies. You will reduce your risk to a long list of diseases, cancers, mental conditions, and obesity as a result of eliminating sugar from your diet. You'll notice drastic positive changes to your health, and you may begin to wonder why you hadn't done this sooner.

There are almost no forms of sugar that provide any health benefits. Your body cannot tell the difference between all of the "healthy" sugars – agave nectar, raw honey, raw sugar, molasses, maple syrup, coconut sugar – and table sugar. The only ones that might be considered, if sweetness is a flavor profile you are looking for in a particular dish, are those that are derived the closest to their natural source. Raw local honey is considered by some to be a reasonable sweetener (but contraindicated for vegans). It's been digested by the bees once already, and it contains a nutritious cocktail of micronutrients, trace minerals, antioxidants and amino acids as well as simple carbohydrates for quick energy. Another source is Grade B maple syrup, which is high in trace minerals such as zinc and manganese, but of course it's more than two-thirds sucrose which makes it suitable for only occasional use. Sweetness, as a flavor profile, is highly overrated. I've grown stevia in my garden, and when you chew on a leaf of it, you will taste its sweetness long after you've spat it out, making it an exercise in aversion therapy.

As you are reading labels in the supermarket aisle, be on the lookout for hidden sugar in your food. See Appendix III for a list of all of the various sugars that are hidden away in modern-day processed foods.

Salt

Salt is not the problem, it's the type of salt. We've become inured to the concept that too much salt in our diets is unhealthy, but as a blanket statement this is patently false. The belief that "salt is unhealthy" is a myth that ranks right up there with "fat makes you fat." Salt has many beneficial properties as an additive to our food. It opens up our taste buds to make food taste better. It stimulates production of the mucosal lining that protects our stomach walls from its harsh acidic environment. Good natural sea salt has trace minerals that are otherwise absent from our diets.

Commercial salt has had all of these trace minerals processed out of it, so that it is over 97% sodium chloride with a little bit of added iodine and some anti-caking agents rounding out the balance. By contrast, natural sea salt is only about 80% sodium chloride, with as many as 75 trace minerals including potassium, magnesium, calcium, sulfur, phosphorus, bromine, boron, zinc, iron, manganese, copper and silicon. Your body uses these minerals in a variety of ways, such as iron and zinc to make some of the enzymes that are involved in metabolism, and calcium and magnesium to promote bone health and cellular metabolism.

Michael Pollan, author of **In Defense of Food: An Eater's Manifesto**, says that "It seems to be a rule of nutritionism that for every good nutrient, there must be a bad nutrient to serve as its foil, the latter a focus for our food fears and the former for our enthusiasms." This is certainly true of salt. Snack foods that rely on large amounts of salt are inherently empty of usable nutrients, while lightly salting your home-prepared dishes with natural sea salt is a simple way to make a remarkably healthy addition to your diet.

We talked earlier about minerals as essential macronutrients. Another word for dietary minerals is electrolytes. We've all heard this term before, but few of us understand what it means. Think of your body's neural pathways as electrical cabling, and know that this cabling is made up of links between atoms of copper, calcium, carbon, zinc, chromium, iron and so on. They help to transfer the specific electrical impulses coming from your brain that enable the rest of your body to react in a certain way; for example, to signal your fingers to turn the page when you've gotten to the bottom of this one, and to provide the mechanical motivation to make them do so. When I mentioned that our bodies are amazing machines, this is one of the things I was referring to.

Vegetarians and Vegans

I am not one to tell people what they should eat (OK, I guess I am), but if you have chosen to go on a vegetarian or vegan diet, I want you to consider that for most people it is an unhealthy food choice. Granted, I don't think anyone should swing to the other end of the spectrum and eat any meat that comes from a Concentrated Animal Feeding Operation (CAFO); even the name itself is quite off-putting. What I would rather see is that more people who consume meat first consider reducing their consumption of meat, and secondly procure the meat that they do eat directly from a farmer or rancher who humanely raises his or her animals in an appropriate manner. Jamming thousands of cows or pigs or chickens together into the tiniest space available is a great way to produce obese, stressed-out meat that is rife with antibiotics, growth hormones and one another's bacteria. I wouldn't come near anything like that, and I hope none of you would, either.

And there's the moral argument that we shouldn't be killing animals for our own convenience. Never mind the fact that we kill plants and eat them, and we kill trees to make the houses we live in, and so on. But let's get off the slippery slope and assume that the moral argument is sound and factually correct. Let's take it several steps further and assume that the whole world wakes up tomorrow and chooses to stop eating all forms of meat, or even stops it in a gradual multiphasic manner. We will be left with billions of cows, chickens, sheep, and goats and so on that

71

we won't use for food anymore. What shall we do with them? Let them run free? Keep them as backyard pets? Slaughter them anyway? I don't have a good answer for that one.

It is possible to get protein and other nutrients from plant sources, but that is not without its own set of problems. Soy, for example, was once considered a reasonable source of plant-based protein, but these days, around 94% of soy produced in America is genetically modified. Soy is also a dangerous hormone disruptor that can create more problems than it resolves. Quinoa is also high in protein, but its production is being scaled up to meet a new global demand, and I fear that it's just a matter of time before the genetic modifiers get their hands on this crop too. It was once a staple for indigenous tribes in South America, and now, due to increased demand, its market value has gone so high that they can no longer afford it unless they grow it for themselves. Certain nutrients, such as Vitamin A, are in their most bioavailable forms when procured from animal sources; the process of creating enzymes required to metabolize Vitamin A has already been done by the animals. It's possible to synthesize Vitamin A from other sources, such as beta-carotene and other carotenoids, but this process is very expensive to the body in terms of the energy required to make the metabolic conversion.

There is also the matter of dietary heritage. If you come from a family in which the last several generations were traditionally vegetarian, it's probably fine that you are a vegetarian as well. A friend of mine hails from Bangalore, in India, and several generations of his family have traditionally been vegetarians, so it makes perfect dietetic sense for him to be vegetarian as well. My ancestors come from northern Europe and Britain, and have eaten meat since time immemorial. Who am I, then, in the course of just my own generation, to suddenly decide to adhere to a strict vegetarian diet and not expect my body to go into revolt?

I actually tried vegetarianism for a few years, and for perhaps the worst reason imaginable: because my girlfriend wanted us to be vegetarians. At the time she was studying acupuncture and Oriental medicine, and most of her classmates chose vegetarianism. So we, admittedly, succumbed to peer pressure and ate a no-meat diet that was heavily weighted towards carbohydrates, things like beans and rice and bagels, and in the two years we lived together we each gained at least twenty pounds. During my studies as a nutritional therapist, a lecturer once asked for a show of hands for those who identified as vegetarian, and no one raised their hands. Then he asked us to raise our hands if we'd ever been vegetarian, and about a third of us had. Empirical data, I know, but remarkable just the same.

Lastly, the people who are not only vegetarians themselves but raise their children as vegetarians are doing severe, perhaps irreparable harm to their children. During a child's formative years, they need nutrients in tremendous amounts and from a variety of sources in order to flourish as they were meant to. People who only feed their children a strict vegetarian diet are, to my mind, in the same category as parents who only feed their children cheap junk food. The motivations may be different, but the harm they are doing to a child's developing body is equally heinous.

How To Eat

Eating is an important part of our innate self-preservation instinct. This is the one thing that we have to do for ourselves; it's not like someone else can eat for us and have that nourishment vicariously enrich our bodies. Nourishing ourselves is a moment when we can be completely self-choosing, and at that choice point we can go in any direction. Some people become the type of person who is always doing things for others - whether it's the family, the job, the social life - so that eating becomes a secondary consideration to the amount of care we provide to others. Once we finally get a chance to sit down and eat, it's in a hurry or is disrupted by having to take care of someone else's needs. We don't take the time to appreciate the fact that we are nourishing ourselves to keep our own physical machine running.

Telling you how to eat makes it sound as if I am telling you how to breathe or walk or make your heart pump blood through your arteries. It's something that seems so natural and instinctive that we never think of how we should be eating. Many of us pay more attention to having proper table manners than we do to what happens to our food once it's made its way into our mouths. Certainly, we all know how to reach for a bit of food, whether with our hands, a fork and knife, chopsticks or a spork. We can accurately size up how much will fit into our mouths with each bite. We know how to chew up our food, tearing it with our incisors, crushing it between our molars, and rolling it between our tongue and palate to break it up until it's small enough to swallow. We know how to keep doing that until we're satiated, or until all the food is gone. But is that really the best way to eat your food?

As mentioned in the previous section, the act of chewing your food is the first step in the assembly line. This is the point at which you have the greatest amount of control over the digestive process. It then becomes imperative for us to learn how we can refine this part of the process as much as possible, in order to ensure that the rest of the workers on your assembly line can do their jobs well by extracting the greatest amounts of nutrients from your food.

Eating should always be treated as a meditation. As in my previous assembly-line analogy, if your mouth is the first stage of the assembly line, the stage prior to that, your brain, is like the auto plant receiving an order to build a car. It's necessary, then, to mentally prepare your self to begin the process of eating. In many cultures, regardless of their faith tradition, it's common before eating a meal together that everyone pauses for a moment, joins in a prayer, or silently asks a blessing. While this might serve to fulfill their spiritual needs, it also prepares the mind to signal the body into digestion. This is a trigger for the autonomic nervous system, an internal control system that acts unconsciously and that regulates basic functions such as breathing, heart rate, digestion, elimination, and even pupillary response and sexual response.

Mindful eating is as much about intention as it is attention. We must teach ourselves how to eat with the fullest intention that we are energizing and healing our bodies in a way that is loving and caring for ourselves. We must also eat with our full attention – noticing the food we are eating and the effects it will have on our bodies. Pay close attention to the food itself. Do you know where it came from? Does it look appealing to you? Who prepared it, and how? How does it taste, and how does each bite feel in your mouth? Is it crunchy, creamy, chewy, coarsely or finely textured, firm or soft? Can you feel bits of it crushing between your molars? Can you tell when a bite of it has been broken down enough to swallow? Do you want more of that, do you want to move on to something else for a moment, or is the whole meal simply not at all palatable to you? Becoming conscious of everything that is happening as you eat is a way of practicing mindful eating, and you will take this practice more and more into every meal you enjoy.

The opposite of mindful eating, of course, is eating mindlessly. When you are distracted during a meal, you not only deny yourself the full enjoyment of your meal, you disengage from the mind-body connection that eating creates. When your body is not in a parasympathetic state, as we'll describe later, your digestion runs at a much slower rate and you are not getting the full nutrient load from what you're eating. Mindful eating is not self-absorbed eating. You should pay close attention to every bit and sip that crosses your lips, certainly, but not at the expense of enjoying a meal with family and friends. Indeed, camaraderie and fellowship are some of the best reasons for breaking bread with others.

Mindful eating helps you learn how to check in with your direct experience when eating. Reconnecting to your direct sensory experience can become the start of an awakening with your food and your eating habits. You may discover that the flavor of common foods can be transformed by bringing a mindfulness practice to the meal.

How does mindful eating change a meal? Pausing and becoming curious focuses the mind. Questions stimulate the mind and create a focus on the bite of food in your mouth. Mindful eating cultivates becoming grounded in the present moment's awareness of eating. If you practice eating more mindfully, you discover that mindfulness may be just the perfect seasoning for any meal.

Mindful eating is self-nurturing. It nourishes not only the body but also the heart, and it becomes something that gets easier and more enjoyable the more you do it. It promotes a better understanding of your true needs, and helps you become aware of your thoughts, feelings, and physical sensations related to eating. By eating with full intention and attention, you reconnect to your body's innate feelings about hunger and satiety by shifting the focus of control from external authorities to your body's inner wisdom.

Ultimately, you will feel more empowered to make healthier choices, bringing acceptance and balance to your life, unlike dieting which can lead to feelings of deprivation. It also opens you to the possibility of freeing yourself from habitual reactive patterns. With practice, mindfulness cultivates the possibility of freeing yourself of reactive, habitual patterns of thinking, feeling and acting.

Acquire the habit of setting down your fork as you take each bite of food. This not only fosters the ability to savor each bite, it gives you time to chew each bite fully to prepare it for its journey of nutritional assimilation. Soon, your friends will all remark on how much less you are eating, how you're always the slowest eater at the table, and ultimately how much better you look. You can share with them about how you've picked up some new techniques that have helped you become more efficient in your eating, or simply smile politely to yourself. This simple technique will be a tremendous help to the workers at the beginning of your assembly line, and even greater help to the workers further down the line.

Lastly, become aware of how you are referring to your food and your new way of eating, with particular regard to the effect it may have on those around you. Chit-chatting about dieting and fat is so commonplace that we often aren't truly aware of the impact it might have on our self-esteem. When you are with friends and family, be especially mindful of your reactions to how others around you talk about eating and body image (e.g. "I'm so fat!" or the "I'm so fat; No you're not" debate). Keep in mind how the words might affect someone else who may be struggling with food issues.

Being fully mindful of your eating is an easy step to take that can help you overcome a longstanding struggle with weight and the management of chronic disease.

When To Eat

When you wake up in the morning, your body hasn't had any new food in a long time, anywhere from ten to perhaps sixteen hours. While you were sleeping, there were several important processes happening in your body. One is a natural detoxification process that occurs during sleep, and as a result, most people tend to head to the bathroom as soon as their feet hit the floor. This process is as natural as can be, because it's your body's way of eliminating the waste that it's collected during the night.

Having something mineral-rich when you first wake up in the morning, such as a handful of nuts or some fruit or even a few grains of sea salt dissolved in a glass of water is a great way to jump-start your body's need to replace those lost minerals. Some will dissolve the sea salt in water, because your body also needs to replace water lost during the night; others will incorporate a tablespoon of raw apple cider vinegar or the juice of half a lemon, and this couldn't be better for awakening your digestive system and preparing it for its day.

We all know that having a full breakfast is the best way to start the day, but many of my clients tell me they can't seem to find the time, the energy, or the motivation to get it together. I ask my clients to send me a three-day food journal which provides me with a snapshot of everything they've had to eat and drink for a three-day period as well as how it made them feel (energized, tired, bloated, happy, nothing, and so on). Some clients reveal that they regularly tend to skip breakfast entirely, or, even worse, they will munch on a store-bought energy bar as they are on their way to work.

I understand that it's difficult to take the time to properly prepare a nutrient-dense breakfast that will sustain you appropriately through the day. Some of us tend to wake up late because we didn't sleep well during the night. When we wake up, we realize that we have to get the kids ready for school, take care of things we didn't take care of the night before, go to the gym or yoga studio before work, or any number of things that take a back seat to watching what we eat. It's understandable to want to just grab something quick and nosh it down in between scurrying from one task to the next. I would like you to consider that this is doing your body a great disservice, and whatever you do manage to eat is not giving you the fullest benefit.

A couple of recommendations I like to make for clients like these is that they get into the practice of making time for themselves in the morning. It can be just a few minutes, a half hour, or however much time you feel you need, but learning to bring your body into the ideal state to receive nourishment is an important habit to develop. If you find you become distracted by the needs of your children, spouse or pets, you can incorporate them into this as it becomes a part of the family routine.

In many cultures and with various faith traditions, it is not uncommon before each meal to say a prayer or ask a blessing. This can become a moment to enter into a parasympathetic state - the calming "rest and digest" state of the autonomic nervous system, which we'll learn more about later – that will bring your body into a more relaxed mode for proper digestion. Turn off the TV, close your laptop, put your phone on silent and just take a moment to be with each other as you are sharing a meal together.[9] Enforcing

---

[9]   I have heard of a recent new thing that people do in restaurants called the "phone stack," and I think it's brilliant. Everyone stacks their cell phones in the middle of the table, and the first person to check for messages or calls has to pick up the tab. If this is what you need to do

this might seem draconian to some members of your family at first, but it will quickly develop into a habit that everyone will look forward to. If you share with them the reason for taking a moment before meals, it will instill in each of them the same practices that they can bring into their lives as they go on about their day and share meals with others. But most importantly, it will consistently help them (and perhaps their fellow diners) to become healthier by switching their digestive systems into a more efficient mode.

Choosing the right place and the right time to eat can be a tall order for some people. You can sit back and think about a peaceful happy place where you envision the food going through your body, blissfully giving in to the tidal surges of peristaltic massage as it breaks down from yummy bites into helpful molecules that are dutifully borne off to the appropriate cells in your body where they can do you the most good. When reality hits, you suddenly realize that you have to leave for work, drop the kids off at school, take them to soccer practice in the afternoon without being late again, and then try to get something to eat for yourself before you head back to the office where it's quieter and you can get a few things accomplished before picking the kids back up again. This is no proper way to eat. Sure, you can let it happen a few times now and then, but when it becomes a part of your regular routine, you leave yourself open for chronic dyspepsia, with all the trickle-down effects it brings.

Small snacks throughout the day are not only beneficial, but encouraged. When you feel hungry, a few bites of something will certainly tide you over, but of course you will want to keep away from processed snack foods and candy bars. Be aware that many of the so-called energy bars are full of processed sugar and refined complex carbohydrates. I've included lists of the various names for hidden sugar in the Appendix to help you find them

---

to bring yourself back into a place of enjoying your food and enjoying the people with whom you are enjoying it, you have my fullest support.

in the lengthy ingredients list, but the best choice is to just go with single-ingredient snacks. Apples, a banana, an orange will all help you through snack time. Another signal for the hunger response is slight dehydration, and so having a glass of water can help resolve your hunger without adding anything that your body doesn't need.

It's important to avoid eating anything within two to four hours before sleeping, assuming you are on what is considered a normal sleeping pattern. If you eat just before sleeping, digestion takes priority over detoxification and overrides the natural detox process. If you happen to eat just before going to bed every once in a while, this is probably not going to be a great problem, but if you develop a natural habit of eating before bedtime you are setting yourself up for a restriction of the natural detoxification process.

Another interesting process that happens during sleep is something called gluconeogenesis. Since you haven't eaten in several hours before sleeping, the body still requires energy to perform all the housekeeping functions that happen while you are sleeping. The liver, which stores glucose in the form of glycogen, converts that back to glucose in a process known as glycolysis. When the liver's glycogen stores are depleted and the body requires more energy than what's been stored, the liver then turns to stored amino acids and fatty acids to convert them into a form of glucose. This happens, on an average night, sometime between the hours of about 1 AM and 3 AM, and if you were to wake up suddenly during the night and palpate your liver, you might find it to be slightly warm to the touch because it's been diligently feeding you from the various nutrients it's kept stored for this purpose.

In addition to choosing the right time of day to eat the right things, you also need to be considerate of the right time of year in which to eat certain foods. We've come to accept the modern concept of the supermarket, with its produce section brimming with all sorts of fruits and vegetables available on a consistent basis throughout the year, as being perfectly normal. We think nothing of buying fresh tomatoes in February or acorn squash in the middle of summer, and indeed many shoppers are now unaware that discrete seasons for various types of produce even exist. The produce they buy in most supermarkets may have been grown in a hothouse the size of a large warehouse, picked before it's fully ripe to prevent bruising during shipment, and then artificially ripened using treatments like nitrogen gas. The end result is a product that looks wonderful on a store shelf but is nearly tasteless and low in actual nutrients. Conversely, whenever I take friends to a farmers market for their first time, often they comment on how the produce may look a little beat-up, bug-bitten, or otherwise different from what they are used to.

Shopping with the seasons has several benefits. When plants are grown within their normal growing season without being artificially induced, they make their way into your kitchen full of vibrant natural flavor and nutrient density. Their cost is lower, not only to you the shopper, but to the environment as well; much out-of-season produce is grown in other countries in the southern hemisphere such as Chile or Australia where the seasons are inverted, and then flown to the U.S. market at a greater cost to the consumer and yielding a lower selling price to the farmer. You will find that buying fresh locally-produced food in season will taste better and be more satisfying. Your body knows that it's eating foods in season, too, based on the hundreds of generations previous to your own that always ate foods in season; indeed, they had no other choice.

Where To Eat

The point in choosing where you should eat, as mentioned earlier, is in repairing to a place where you can bring your self into a parasympathetic state. Creating a place for your self, alone or with others, is an ideal way to bring your body into a relaxed state that will promote optimal digestion. You may only have this special place for the duration of your meal, but it's important to make it your own for the time being. Invite those who are eating with you into that place to utilize their energy in a way that can bring your self into a calmer state.

This may be difficult to achieve since our modern lives often seem to have us bouncing from one place to the next, often without much warning and often in a self-directed manner. Let's say a project lands on your desk mid-morning with a note from your boss saying something like this:

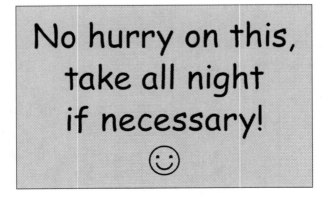

There go your lunch plans. Before you know it, you've worked into the wee small hours and ended up having your supper from the vending machine again, but, doggone it, you nailed that project and had it waiting on your boss's desk first thing in the morning. Stuff happens, and when it does happen, on occasion, your body can quickly recover from it. It's important, though, to learn to take extra time for your self so that, even when life hands you unexpected things like huge work projects or having to shuttle the kids from softball practice to band rehearsals on the same night, you learn to develop the skills to bring your self to a peaceful state for eating. When all around you is utter chaos, you can take a moment and clear out a space that is just for you.

Consider this: a rabbit is being chased through the forest by a fox. The rabbit manages to escape by ducking down a convenient rabbit hole. The rabbit is safe from the fox, but still has a great deal of nervous energy coursing through its little rabbit body. It is not uncommon for the rabbit to just sit there and shake itself vigorously, in an effort to rid itself of the fear energy and being itself back into a calm and relaxed state. You can do the same thing when you are being chased by the foxes in your life. Once you realize that you've reacted to something, and that something has come and gone, create some movement with your body to shake off the strong feelings, usually feelings of fear, and offer yourself a couple of deep breaths to help restore your peaceful energy and create relaxation for your self.

This may seem like another tall order that this book is handing you, and for some it might seem impossible with kids pulling at you and the dog barking and the TV yapping and any number of other outside distractions taking you away from your happy place. You may feel as though you're reading from a work of fiction, but bringing yourself in to a peaceful state can turn out to be pretty simple, once you get into the habit of doing it.

The best way to calm down your world is to start with calming your self. You have little to no influence on the people in your life, but you have complete control over how you react to them. If you find that the same buttons keep getting pushed by the same people or situations, take a moment to think about whose buttons they are in the first place. The ultimate conclusion is that they are all yours, of course, which means that you can disable them or at least put them on a delay so you can handle the button-pushers with a touch more serenity.

Regardless of life's chaotic tendencies, bringing your self to a state of peace and calm before eating does your body, mind and spirit a tremendous amount of good. We touched on the autonomic nervous system previously, but now is a good time to talk about it in greater depth.

The autonomic nervous system is regulated by the hypothalamus, an organ that is nestled deep inside the brain. It controls several bodily functions that are grouped into two classes:

Sympathetic ("Fight or Flight")

- Enhances blood flow to skeletal muscles by as much as 1200%
- Dilates bronchioles in the lungs to increase blood oxygenation
- Increases heart rate to promote circulation to skeletal muscles
- Creates energy in the skeletal muscles by releasing glucose
- Dilates the pupils of the eyes to increase distant vision
- Slows down digestion and inhibits peristalsis
- Constricts all intestinal sphincters and the urinary sphincter

Parasympathetic ("Rest and Digest")

- Dilates intestinal blood vessels to promote digestion and nutrient absorption
- Relaxes the bronchioles when demand for oxygen has diminished
- Slows heart rate to normal or even slightly lowered levels
- Slows down the release of glucose into the bloodstream
- Constricts the pupils to accommodate better near vision
- Stimulates salivary gland secretion and accelerates peristalsis

In both states, there are a lot of things happening all at once and they tend to be mutually exclusive. When one organ or system is put on alert in one state, it becomes relaxed in the other. It's clear from this information that we always want to bring ourselves into the parasympathetic "rest and digest" state before we eat a meal. The inner core of your brain, including the hypothalamus, doesn't know the difference between what you're doing and what stimuli your body is receiving, so it can't distinguish whether you are being chased by a buffalo, or whether you are just scarfing down a cheeseburger while zig-zagging through rush hour traffic. In either event, your food will not get digested any time soon, and until you do come to a parasympathetic state the food will just sit in your belly and turn yucky.

Here's something to imagine, or you can try it in real life if you'd care to. The next time you have dinner, set aside one portion of everything you've made including the beverage you paired it with. Put it all into a blender, and then collect a large mouthful of saliva and expectorate that into the blender as well. Blend the contents thoroughly, and then leave it to rest at 98.6°F (37°C) for several hours. This will give you a good idea of what happens to undigested food in your stomach. It just sort of sits there and doesn't get digested, because digesting enzymes aren't being secreted into it in any quantity, and you end up with a huge mess that just gets thrown out later.

Let's amplify a portion of the earlier discussion we had on the digestive process. After your stomach has held onto its contents for a while, it sends everything down the line bit by bit, whether it's done a spectacular job of breaking everything down or not. If you are eating while you're in a sympathetic state, your stomach hasn't been given a full chance to completely digest your food, but when its time in the stomach is up, it goes on down the intestinal assembly line regardless. The workers down the line - enteric biota or "gut bugs" – have to either work a lot harder to extract nutrients from this mess or they simply will not be able to do a complete job, and here's where your trouble begins. After just a few hours, proteins putrefy, fats rancidify, and carbohydrates ferment. This goes a long way in explaining a lot of the gassiness, bloating and rumbling noises (the old "organ recital") that you notice after certain meals, especially those high in carbohydrates that have not been well chewed.

If this is a common occurrence for you, consider your mental state as well as any outside disruptions you may have experienced while you were eating. Did you do a quick "grab and go" lunch again? Were you eating in the car while rushing from one appointment to another? Did you pig out during a football game or a scary movie? All of these things contribute to poor digestion, and a habit of eating under these conditions leads to a wide spectrum of possible disorders that would be enough to fill another book, in and of itself.

Apart from being mindful of where you are when you are eating, consider another "where" possibility. Do you know where your food came from? Most of us don't, and I'd wager that the majority of that group never even thinks about it. Very few of us live on farms any more, and almost none of us have anything more than a small garden by our homes. We gather the bulk of our food at a local supermarket, not reaped from our own soil or butchered on our own ranch. As a society, we just don't do that anymore. I have met many people who have given up on knowing anything about where their food comes from, and I am frequently being called out as the "gourmet chef" among my friends just because I can butterfly a chicken breast; indeed, so few of them have even considered butterflying a chicken breast themselves that the simple act of cutting a piece of meat along its X axis seems curiously exotic.

I do the majority of my grocery shopping at my local farmers market. I'm glad I live in a city where there are four farmers markets that stay open year-round, and during the summer months there is a farmers market somewhere in town every day of the week. I get a deep satisfaction in handing my money over directly to the person who produced the food I plan to eat. I appreciate that there's no middle-man involved, and they are getting a fair price for some very hard work that I don't care to do myself. I also get to ask them questions about the food and how it was created. What breed of hogs or chickens or goats are these from? Where is your farm located, and what are the soil conditions? When did you catch these fish? They almost always know enough to talk your ear off about it, and I'm always eager to learn something new.

Buying organic at these markets is almost a given, although it's not necessarily true in all cases, so you can ask them how or if they use pesticides and artificial fertilizers if you want. Though I'm not a farmer, I've learned of some innovative techniques of companion planting that keep bugs and rodents from spoiling your crop without having to resort to spraying. Start raising your curiosity around your food and its origins. Your body will thank you.

Why To Eat

Certainly, eating and creating nourishment is one of the basic survival instincts in which all organisms get to participate. But there are reasons to eat, such as to strengthen your body and stave off starvation, and there are reasons not to eat, such as to avoid overeating and to conserve some of the available food for later.

Researchers have recently discovered a new type of hormone called leptin. The word 'hormone' come from an ancient Greek word meaning 'impetus,' and hormones are used as messengers from one organ to another carrying a message that it's time to do something. The leptin hormone is unusual because it is not stored and secreted as part of an endocrine or exocrine gland. It's actually kept in adipose tissue - body fat - and its purpose is to start and stop the feast-or-famine response. When the body has not had enough dietary intake for a long enough period of time, the fat cells start releasing leptin into the bloodstream so that it is carried to the hypothalamus, which then signals other parts of the body to begin looking for something to eat. This is how your mind controls whether you need to go gather some more roots and berries, stake out a herd of bison, or turn off at the next exit to find a nice restaurant.

Once you've gotten that strong leptin signal and found something to eat the release of leptin decreases, activating the satiation response and turning off the hunger response. Before long you just don't feel like eating very much anymore, and you may feel as though your tummy is full but it's really because your brain has received the signal that you've had enough for now. You would think that if you are obese, because you possess more adipose tissue you should have a more responsive leptin pathway, but this just leads to confusion. Although leptin reduces the hunger response, obese individuals generally exhibit a higher circulating concentration of leptin due to their higher percentage of body fat. This actually leads to a resistance to the leptin signal, much as Type II diabetics develop a resistance to insulin to regulate their blood sugar. The elevated levels of leptin fail to control hunger and regulate weight because the leptin receptors in the brain become indifferent to the increased leptin signals. Your body's leptin stores have cried "Wolf!" a few too many times.

This may all sound very four-eyed and technical, and I urge you to research it further if you'd like because I feel that knowing more about this can help you to understand why and how hunger happens. If you are daydreaming about doughnuts, instead of toddling down to the local bakery or even the vending machine, consider that your body may just be responding to a release of leptins. There are many ways to overcome this response, but one of the simplest ways is to just have a glass of water.

In his book **Your Body's Many Cries For Water**, Dr. Fereydoon Batmanghelidj states that our brain is only 2% of our body mass but accounts for over 25% of our body's water stores. Brain cells are up to 85% water, and when these cells begin to run dry, just as in my earlier analogy of rivers and creeks and streams, they do not perform at their best and it's possible for them to either become confused or resistant to the hormonal messages they are meant to receive. Maintaining proper hydration, meaning water and not just fluids of any old type, is critical in keeping this neural communication pathway open and working properly.

Wanting to eat when your body is really just thirsty is one indicator that your internal messaging is all wonky. There are many other reasons, such as that you have been using food as a coping mechanism for strong emotional feelings. If you just had a stroke of good luck, you might feel like indulging in a treat. If you're sad or lonely, nobody will understand you like food does. Angry? You might take out your frustrations with a knife and fork. Turning to food for emotional reasons won't resolve the underlying issues.

Try tracking what you eat by creating a food journal, as I recommend my clients to do. Include the time of day, what you ate or drank, and how you felt at the time. Be brutally honest with your self and be sure to log everything. No one needs to see this but you (and perhaps your health practitioner, if you choose to share it), but doing this lifts the veil of secrecy and shame that you might feel about using food to act out. You'll begin to recognize connections that you hadn't noted before, such as eating when you are lonely or angry, or sneaking a snacky treat when nobody is looking. Once you find this connection and reveal it for what it is, you can begin to create a new awareness around knowing when you are "eating your emotions."

Perhaps sometimes you are not eating when you're emotional, but just out of sheer boredom. Eating might seem like a good thing to do when there's nothing else to do, whether you graze while you're at work or at home, on lazy weekends, or even by entertaining yourself with a lavish dinner out. Eating only occupies some of the time, though, and then you have to do something with the rest of your time. Think of it like having an itch on your arm. You scratch to relieve the itch, but that's not what scratching an itch does. It simply replaces the feeling of itchiness on the surface of your skin with another feeling, so your brain quickly forgets that your skin was itchy. If you find long and frequent periods of boredom in your life, it should come as a friendly indicator for you to discover and follow your passion.

Consider something that you've always wanted to do and then start focusing your energy toward that. Remember that where the mind goes, energy follows, so if your mind follows your passions, then your energy will go there too.

Do you ever find yourself in a situation where you are eating because other people are eating? I'd say we all do from time to time. Everyone at work wants to go out to the new Mega Burger for lunch, and you're thinking of the carrot sticks you brought from home that pale in comparison to fun-filled camaraderie, endless baskets of fries, and wanton disregard of your satiation level. You want to fit in because everyone else is going, and now you look on those carrot sticks as prison bars. It's fine to break out once in a while, be with the crowd and enjoy a great time, but become aware of what foods you are drawn to and what you should order. By all means, I encourage you to enjoy sparkling conversation and high times as you effortlessly choose a lighter meal than the others are having, and just have water to drink, please. No ice.

There are special occasions in which food is offered as a part of the celebration, and certainly this is a custom as old as time itself. The Bible is filled with feasts of thanksgiving, the Passover Seder, the feeding of the multitudes and so on, and you can find similar stories of celebratory feasts throughout nearly every type of historical account. If you live with a large extended family, or work in a big office with lots of coworkers, it's always someone's birthday, anniversary, baby shower or who-knows-what. When I worked in Corporate America, at every meeting some well-intentioned coworker would bring in a box of doughnuts, and we often had pizza ordered in just because it was Friday or because we were working on a deadline.

When I was with Microsoft for ten years, we had a tradition to celebrate your job anniversary by bringing in a bowl of M&Ms, with one pound for every year you'd worked there. I was there ten years, and I stopped honoring that custom after the first few years. It wasn't just the logistics of schlepping in ten pounds of M&Ms and then expecting people to eat it all for you; it was the temptation of so much candy within easy reach. It took little effort for me to eat out of boredom, emotion, or just the habit of instinctively grabbing some nearby food and putting into my mouth. Celebrations should be about the celebrants, and the food should be secondary, but we seem to have lost that message along the way.

Maybe you always eat at specific times of the day, without stopping to think whether you are actually hungry. I had once hired a man who would completely stop his work at noon every day, regardless of how important the task at hand was or who else was depending on him to finish his work. That may be an extreme case, but when the clock on the wall tells you to eat, resist its tyranny and check in to see whether you really are hungry, or whether you're just reacting to an old habit that says you can only eat certain meals at certain times of the day. If you've checked in and, sure enough, you're hungry because it's been several hours since you've had anything, eat. But first teach yourself to check in and see if your current hunger pangs meet the above-mentioned criteria of emotion, boredom, proximity, opportunity, and so on.

Sometimes you'll come across food that is free or unavoidably cheap. Free samples at the grocery store are a good example of this, as are all-you-can-eat buffets and buy-one-get-one-free deals. These are a great chance for you to toss your diet and your willpower out the window and think only of your food budget. Don't give in, or at least loiter at the section of the buffet that has salads and fresh fruits.

Everyone knows a "food pusher," the one who always wants others to eat with them, and to whom saying no is difficult. We all want to be a people pleaser, especially in the giving and receiving of an offering of food. It's hard to turn down something that is skillfully created and lovingly prepared just for you, but you can easily just assert that you are dieting or simply not hungry at the moment. At the very least, taking just a small portion will be considered polite, and the richer the food, the smaller the portion you should take.

Then there's the Clean Plate Club, and coming from a large family I can certainly understand this as a reason to overeat beyond the stage at which your body's natural leptin signals tell you to stop. The well-meaning lessons about starving children in faraway lands or finishing your vegetables because they're good for you are certainly compelling, but if you are full you should just stop eating and save the rest for later. In some cultures, a clean plate means that you were not served enough to eat and would like some more, and if you are dining in the home of people who come from those cultures, be aware of this custom or be prepared to overeat.

You can learn to gauge yourself throughout your meal as to how full you feel, and there's certainly no need to scrape every last ort from your plate (as we used to say, "Send the dishwasher home!"). Try using a smaller plate, or, at a restaurant, there's no shame to ask for a half-order if they can offer that. And become friends with leftovers. When I have clients who tend to skip breakfast because there's no time to cook in the morning, I suggest they consider having leftovers for breakfast.

If you really want to know why you are eating, besides just being hungry, let your self know what true hunger feels like. If you think about it, when was the last time you went for an entire day without eating? Doing this sort of mini-fast can help you to check in and see why your leptin receptors keep ringing the dinner bell. During this time, distract your thoughts of eating with other work, such as a project that requires deep concentration. Whether this is at your job or as part of a hobby that you enjoy, when you focus your mind on anything other than food you will find that time has gone by quickly and the feelings of hunger you had before are quickly offset by other thoughts. I've made a simple guideline so you can know at what level of hungriness you are feeling at any given time, and you can use this in your food journal as a form of shorthand.

Hunger Level	Signs and Sensations
1	Famished, dizzy, weak, trembling
2	Very hungry, cranky, low energy, tummy growling
3	Rather hungry, stomach rumbling a little
4	Just starting to feel hungry
5	Neither hungry nor full
6	Pleasantly full, could take just another bite
7	Mildly uncomfortable
8	Completely satisfied
9	Very uncomfortable, stomach aches
10	So full you want to vomit for relief

SECTION III

Healthy

When, in disgrace with fortune and men's eyes,
I all alone beweep my outcast state,
And trouble deaf heaven with my bootless cries,
And look upon myself, and curse my fate,
Wishing me like to one more rich in hope,
Featur'd like him, like him with friends possess'd,
Desiring this man's art and that man's scope,
With what I most enjoy contented least;
Yet in these thoughts myself almost despising,
Haply I think on thee, and then my state,
Like to the lark at break of day arising
From sullen earth, sings hymns at heaven's gate;
For thy sweet love remember'd such wealth brings
That then I scorn to change my state with kings.
                    William Shakespeare, Sonnet 29

Wellness is a choice. It's a gift we purchase for ourselves and receive joyfully. Each meal is a new beginning as we take the opportunity to heal our bodies and change our lives. Wellness is a side effect of the process we take to get from a state of neglect or indifference to a state of deep self-care. By the time we've arrived at this stage, we know most of the things we need to do to restore and maintain good health. We may slip up a time or two, but our bodies have become stronger and better prepared to withstand physical, emotional, and spiritual stress. From here, we can move into a place of continual nourishment of our bodies, minds and spirits. We've turned away from the things that once interested us because we know that they no longer serve us well. We've created a new life for ourselves that suits our own bioindividual needs.

We look to the teachings of our chosen faith traditions that remind us that our bodies are a temple to honor and serve our Creator. We have chosen to not pollute that temple with things that will get in the way of our honoring and our service. Others may scoff and ask us if we've gone on the latest fad diet, but we've really just made radical changes to our way of thinking in order to make room for the inevitable change that naturally fills and fulfills our lives. Old habits have slipped away from us, and though the motivation behind them may still exist, we've changed the focus of that motivation into new ways that generate greater levels of health and happiness for us. We can choose from a wide variety of healthful foods that will nourish us fully. We drink water in sufficient quantities to enable and sustain a higher quality of living. We exercise regularly in ways that are appropriate for our physical condition. We replenish our bodies and restore our souls. We actively reduce stressful situations in our lives. We keep our minds active and endeavor to always learn new things. We experience the abundant joy of living, we pursue greater meaning in our lives, and we allow ourselves to relax and find peace.

Not all of us are born healthy. Nobody's perfect. As mentioned earlier, with regard to bioindividuality, we all have our strengths and our weaknesses. Some of us may even have conditions that are difficult to overcome, and in hearing these words might think that becoming perfectly well is simply not something that is available to them. They would be right, and the same thing can be said of all of us. We are imperfect beings, so expecting perfection is like Don Quixote tilting at windmills. We try, sometimes even going to the extremes of reconstructive surgery, starvation diets, or grueling workout regimens. At some point we have to accept that we are enough just as we are. We can - and should - continue to push up to and against our perceived limits, but at some point we must also take a moment to appreciate who we are and how far we've come to get to where we are in this moment.

What Optimal Health Feels Like

For many of us, we've allowed ourselves to get so far into a condition of poor health that we have come to accept our condition as the "new normal," as just a part of growing older. We become resigned to the fact that there's nothing we can do about it. We feel as though we just have to accept our fate and deal with it. It's not so bad, anyway, once you get used to it, right?

A growing number of people have decided that this is not how their lives are going to turn out. They cannot completely reverse the effects of growing older, but they can mitigate or even eliminate the problems they have developed as a result of a poor diet. They seek for themselves a newer way of living, a newer course of action to divert their lives away from one of inevitable deterioration and towards a life filled with happiness, lightness, and the freedom to continue to enjoy the things they did when they were younger. They are ordinary people like you and me, far removed from celebrities and know-it-all authors of self-help books. They lace up their running shoes one foot at a time, same as you and me, and they go out there every day and try to make a difference in their lives.

For their efforts, they have developed a renewed energy and stamina. They find that they don't get tired so easily. They sleep through the night and awake refreshed. They are able to spend more and better time with their kids and grandkids. Their bodies feel lighter, and simple movements have become easier. Aging, physical decay and death await us all, but these are people who work hard to fend off that eventuality for as long as possible. Each of us gets the exact number of hours in each day, though we all get our own allotment of days that we get to be here. Some people see that as a challenge, an empty bucket to be filled up with as much activity, experiences, and people as possible before they reach their ultimate end.

I don't have any children of my own, but I have got parents. Had, that is, until they both passed away in 2011; first Mom, then Dad a few months later. So, speaking from the place of a childless individual, I'll say that the most important thing parents can do for their children is to inspire them. My parents both died of preventable lifestyle-based conditions. Their death certificates list the exact causes of their deaths, but they both essentially just checked out of life long before life was done with them. It seemed that, after raising five boys into grown men, their work here on Earth was complete and there was nothing left for them to do. They invested in a pair of comfortable recliners, signed up for the premium cable TV package, and sat and watched as the world went by them. If I sound bitter and angry, I am. It makes me furious that their lifestyle choices robbed me of my parents so early in life. Mom was only 73 and Dad was 77. They'd met in their hometown of Bryan, Texas, and were married for over fifty years until untimely death did them part, and their remains were returned back to Bryan for burial.

Still, they inspired me greatly. I've listed them in the acknowledgements for teaching me that cooking is fun, but they also inspired me to not let my life turn out as theirs did. I'd foreseen a similar mindset looming in my own future, and after their deaths I found that my own decline and mortality suddenly became very authentic. Would the end come to me in my mid-fifties, alone in a small apartment in Seattle, or would it be several decades later, after enjoying a beautiful life well spent with incredible friends, wild adventures, and glorious moments of exquisite beauty? I chose the latter, and I wanted to take this life lesson and use it to broaden my passion for nutritional health and mindful wellness to as many people as possible, in hopes that they will choose not to suffer a fate similar to that of my late parents.

Getting Over Your Self

There is a phrase that I've learned that sounds stern and off-putting at first, but when I finally examined it and took its meaning to heart, it put everything in a nutshell for me. In order to begin creating change in our lives, we need to change ourselves first. Absolutely nothing can happen to make significant changes in our thinking and our daily habits until we properly prepare ourselves to become willing to make changes. Change is inevitable and unavoidable, and it enables growth, vitality, and health. The entire universe is constantly changing every second. Even though we look up at the stars, they seem to always be in the same place every night, but they aren't. This reminds me of a passage by Kurt Vonnegut Jr. in his novel **The Sirens Of Titan**, "Every passing hour brings the Solar System forty three thousand miles closer to Globular Cluster M13 in Hercules – and still there are some misfits who insist that there is no such thing as progress."

So it is within your body. You were once an infant, then a child, a teenager, a young adult and so on to the stage at which you find yourself now. You've been changing all of your life, even though you feel that you have always been the same person, and in many ways you are. You may feel the same even though your body has been constantly changing, but consider that you are holding on to the past without an awareness of the present. Becoming aware of your present is the initial stage to accepting change as an important and non-negotiable part of your life cycle.

Within your mind, you must learn to accept that change is required in order for you to move your life forward. There are people who actually prefer to remain stuck in the past, looking back on times that may have been happier or that held a special appeal to them. Keeping your mind cemented in the past prevents you forever from moving forward, and leaves you grasping at the ghosts of the past that have long since evaporated. Dreaming of a perfect future is also fleeting, and the future owes us no favors. So that leaves us with the present. At the present, I am sitting somewhere cozy writing this book, and in your present moment you are likely seated somewhere cozy reading it. If you're not sitting someplace cozy, you probably have the freedom and ability to move someplace else where you can be more comfortable. Go on, move to a cozier spot, if you'd like. Put your feet up. Now pat yourself on the back, because you just changed your present condition. It can be as easy as that: you were not comfortable with your present condition, and so you made a conscious choice to change.

We all tend to gravitate toward comfort foods, the foods that we ate when we were younger that were good for us, that tasted good to us, or that were given to us as a reward for being good boys and girls. Growing up mostly in the South, the comfort food we had wasn't necessarily the best for us, but it was made lovingly and offered thoughtfully. Using food as a reward system is an ages-old keystone of parenting, but the end result is that we tend to carry that tradition into our adult years. A little snack or piece of candy when we are young evolves into binge eating and sugar addiction in our later years. As mentioned before, our bodies are wondrously resilient and capable of recovering from occasional damage, but decades of abuse will inevitably take its toll.

We need to learn how to get out of our own way and shed the romantic view of our past that we have carried into our adult years. We must condition ourselves to become more open to making changes within ourselves, with the understanding that these

105

changes are necessary to strengthen us and heal us. We need to accept that anything and everything we've come to know about food might be wrong, and that taking on new habits and new ideas just might steer us back along the road to optimal health.

At the beginning of this chapter I'd promised to share with you a phrase that will help you to make the changes that you need to make, and here it is:

GET OVER
YOUR SELF!

As I promised, this may land on you as blunt and unforgiving, abrupt and arrogant, but it's actually a precise and important truth. Until we can get over our selves, we'll still continue to go down the same paths as before, making the same mistakes we always seem to make, compensating for those mistakes as we've taught ourselves to do, and ultimately moving not one inch forward in our lives. The realization that you need to get over your self inflicts serious damage to your old ways of thinking, and therefore creates new openings into new possibilities for growth and progress.

Just as a hatchling pecks away at the shell that confines it and prevents it from further growth, so must we destroy the shell that's kept us inside our old ways of thinking so we can create whole universes of possibility. Getting over your self opens up new pathways for empowerment, ultimately creating a new life for your self that greatly surpasses the predictable. A fully predictable and almost certain future comes out of your past, but by making change a tool that you can use to open up a space for new possibilities in the present, your future suddenly becomes nothing but possibility.

The edict to get over your self is not intended as another opportunity to clobber yourself in self-directed resentment or incessant rumination of things you "woulda coulda shoulda" done. Nobody likes guilt trips. I offer this to you as a way of examining your life from a new perspective, of seeing what had driven you to make the choices you had made in the past, and, once you've cleared those out of the way, to look at other possibilities as a conscious choice going forward. This is not just me angrily shouting, "Get over your self!" at you, but rather it's you saying it to your self in your own voice. Say it gently, lovingly, with an air of self-care and even with a hint of giddy excitement over the new possibilities that will be revealed to you.

The only time that change can happen is in this moment right now. Yesterday is gone, and it won't come back. Tomorrow isn't here yet, so that's out, too. Certainly you should make plans for your future and hope that the future works out according to your best-laid plans, but we all know what happens to plans when we fail to predict the unpredictable. So that leaves us in the present, the only point in time in which we always exist. If you recently moved your seating accommodation to something you've found to be more comfortable, you changed your present because your past became uncomfortable.

When I learned to get over myself, and constantly reminded myself to do so, at first it was difficult. It was hard to hear, and it merged with the chorus of negative statements I'd been carrying around inside my head. When someone finally spelled it out to me in a manner similar to what I've described here, I was finally able to see what I'd been doing. I had the epiphany that my best thinking had only gotten me as far as where I was at that time. I had ended up in a hospital bed, deathly ill and almost incapable of taking care of myself at the tender age of fifty-one, and I see it as the direct result of not being able to get over my self and take direct action. I ultimately made a selfish choice, and I use that term with no fear of egocentric self-seeking. I chose myself. I had decided that I was important enough to take care of, despite all my years of doing whatever I wanted and not caring much about the outcome. Once I reached the stage where I learned that I needed to get over myself, to transcend my ego, I felt as if I had been liberated from everything I'd been carrying around from my past. The sensation of true freedom was exhilarating.

So try it. The next time you come across a difficult decision in your life, whether it's your career choices, your relationship choices, or just when you go grocery shopping, take a moment to go inside your self and see what stands in your way of making a choice that serves your best interests. Certainly, there may be external things blocking you from making a selfish choice, and there are some things you can directly affect while other things may leave you completely powerless to change them. But the practice of getting over your self enables you to look at how much of your self is doing the disempowerment. You are the only person in the world over which you have complete control, so check in to see what you *can* control to create the change you want to make in your life. You might find that you are the only one who is standing in your way. Your will to change eventually becomes greater than your ego's desire to be comfortable.

This is one of those processes where you end up getting out of it what you've put into it. If you finish this book and think to yourself, "Meh, I didn't get that much out of it," I'd like you to consider this: how much of your self you have put into it? If you put a hundred percent of your energy into wanting to make significant change in your life, you will be amazed at what your mind can bring you to do, even before you've finished this book. The principles I mention here are universal and exist in a wide variety of both spiritual and secular teaching.

In the Taoist tradition they say, "Where the mind goes, energy follows," and that's quite true. If your mind keeps going to food choices that you know are unhealthy, for example, you'll keep putting your energy toward those choices and getting the same results; the same food that you know is bad for you will keep showing up every time you unpack your grocery bag.

If you work hard to consciously retrain your mind to make different choices, your energy will begin to follow that path instead. You will instinctively steer away from the harmful choices you used to make. You will awaken to the fact that your mind is capable of creating infinite possibilities. You may even become inspired to write a book about your experience, and I sincerely hope that you do. There are over seven billion stories to be told, and yours is one of them.

What To Do If It's Not Working

Regardless of the type of changes you need to make, you will find that it will either get better or get worse. When you start making radical changes to your diet, for example, you can experience any of several common body reactions. If you have been living for years on a steady diet of "whatever," your body has been slightly modified to become accustomed to that sort of diet. Doing a sudden and sharp U-turn in the opposite direction, dietetically speaking, causes your body to go into revolt. Your body expects a steady conveyor belt of one type of food, and if you start introducing something completely different into it you can expect a different set of results from your digestive system. When you think about it, this explains how things like traveler's diarrhea, the so-called "Montezuma's Revenge," works. It's often blamed on unsanitary food handling when, in fact, much of it is just due to an abrupt change in diet based on the local offerings versus what you can get back home.

Here are three ways that your body can react to abrupt changes in your diet, what you can expect, and what to do when they occur. In all cases, if you are under the care of a professional, they should be notified immediately of any significant changes.

- **Healing reaction** - Your body is beginning to get better, although it might not seem that way at first. You may experience a slight or temporary escalation of your symptoms; they may seem to get worse before they start to get better. That's just your body waging a fierce battle against the forces of evil pathogens, and you've been giving it all the ammunition it needs to win. This is a therapeutic change called retracing, and it is part of Hering's Law of Cure, which comes from a 19th-century text on homeopathy[10]. Hering's Law states that: "All healing occurs from within out, from the head down, and in the reverse order in which the symptoms have appeared." So, as your body begins to heal, it releases the toxins and other elements that it's held onto that are associated with a disease or condition, and as those are leaving your body they might cause some disturbance on their way out. Hang in there, stick with your treatment protocol, and let it ride its course. You are actually getting healthier. For example, when you have a cold or flu, one symptom is a low-grade fever, which is your body's way of raising the basal body temperature in an attempt to make an inhospitable environment for viruses and bad bacteria. This is perfectly natural and normal, if a bit uncomfortable.

- **Digestive reaction** - You may feel a brief bout of upset stomach, nausea, heartburn, excess gassiness, bloating, constipation, diarrhea, or any combination of the above including everything all at once. Again, it's your body's way of evicting the bad pathogens and replacing them with beneficial bacteria cultures. In this process you can expect a little tumult in your tummy. If it becomes too severe, turn to your healthcare provider for further advice, but just riding it out for a day or two might be what they tell you to do. Avoid taking antibiotics unless you are sure that you might have been exposed to any foodborne

---

[10] "Rise and Progress of Homeopathy"; Hering, Constantine; Philadelphia 1834

pathogens that could be causing the problem. This is a side issue and not necessarily caused by the change in diet. And of course, with any introduction of antibiotics you should follow it up with a regimen of pre- and probiotics to reintroduce good bacterial cultures in the wake of a regimen of indiscriminate antibiotics.

- **Allergic or sensitivity reaction** - Stop what you are doing immediately and contact your healthcare provider! You might have uncovered a previously undetected allergy or sensitivity that was not known before, when you were on your "whatever" diet. The most common food allergens are wheat, dairy, soy, nuts, and eggs, but you can develop a sensitivity to just about anything. This can be serious and might even be life-threatening, so I cannot stress its gravity enough. Start a conversation with your healthcare provider about another protocol, because the one you're on right now isn't going to work.

Whenever you have food cravings, your body might just be telling you that you have nutrient deficiencies and is dropping a hint that you need to find a way to resolve them. The problem is that the signal gets mixed up by some of the messages, especially with all the confusing advertising messages that you've received throughout your life. Instead of instinctively choosing the best possible and most nutrient-dense food choices, you are stampeding to the fridge or pantry for a quick fix. This is not a gender-specific thing and happens throughout one's life. We all get this. To help you learn to make better choices, I've included a chart of common food cravings, what deficiencies they represent, and what you can choose instead that will help you to overcome the cravings. Go to Appendix III to learn more about this.

Sometimes we might lack the willpower on our own to create the change we need to make in our lives. This is when it's time to call a friend for help. Tell them you are reading this amazing book by a brilliant new author, and he says a lot of the right things but you just don't know if you can go it alone. Clearly, you need to enlist the aid of a confederate, someone who can understand your situation and listen to your fears without judging. Make it a challenge between the two of you, because it might just be that she or he wanted to get some help as well, but you were the bolder one who had the gumption to actually ask for help. You will find great support in working with someone else as you go through this. Not only will it give you the benefit of support that only a friend can provide, but you will enrich your own life by sharing your support with them.

What To Do If It Is Working

Keep doing what you're doing! You might have just found the Golden Path to Optimal Health, and the items you've taken out of your diet combined with the new things you're eating seem to be the perfect combination for you. Remember what I had mentioned earlier about bioindividuality, that what works great for one person may be harmful to another and have no effect at all on someone else. Perfecting an individual nutritional plan requires a certain amount of tinkering to get things just right, so one important life skill you'll need to embrace is patience. Not only will you end up going down the wrong nutritional rabbit-hole a time or two, but in the meantime life will continue to happen to you. Perhaps an office birthday party or a lavish anniversary dinner might make you forget your body's special needs momentarily, and you may even pay the price the day after, if not sooner. It's OK if you slip up like that, but you'll need to catch yourself soon enough that you don't stray too far into eating the things you're trying to avoid.

You will also come to your own level of homeostasis regarding your attitudes around food. By the time healing has begun to set in, you might give in to the urge to become an amateur nutritionist and start instructing all your friends on what they should and should not eat. I must admit that I fell into this myself early in my career. I became the go-to guy about anything to do with food, and I gladly handed out advice as freely as it was asked; sometimes even more so. When I went out to dinner with friends they would all want to know what I was ordering before making

114

up their own minds, and when I told them what I was planning to order, some would quickly return to the menu with a change of heart. I've decided, outside of my practice, to let people do whatever they want and to generally keep my opinions to myself. If they really want to know what I think about what they eat and its effects on their unique physical condition, I may still have some appointment times available.

Creating and Accumulating Healthy Energy

Optimal health goes far beyond just eating the right foods and avoiding the bad ones. It's more than maintaining a high level of alertness around what your body is doing with the food you've eaten, and what it's doing for you. The bigger picture is more about getting back in touch with your body and learning how it reacts to everything you do with it. Once you have gotten the knack of making the right food choices, you will notice that your daily energy level increases. You no longer wake up still tired, you don't feel like having a nap in the afternoon, and you can continue the things you enjoy doing most well into the late evening.

We all love how great we feel when our energy level is high, and energy is a good marker of our overall health. Here are some ideas that can help you to develop and accumulate more energy, even at those times when you feel like your energy is at an all-time low; especially at those times. It's fine to just pick one of these and start there, and then incorporate more of these practices as you become empowered and inspired to do so.

Enrich Your Energy With Nutritious Food

We've talked about this through most of the book, but it bears repeating so much that it tops this list. We are in a society where we've become addicted to foods that don't really serve our energy, to the point that we can't even recognize it for what it is and what it's doing to us. A diet of processed foods, with their additives and colorings and preservatives, robs us of our energy and leaves us feeling briefly satiated but ultimately unfulfilled and unhealthy. Focus on eating *real* food instead - you know, the kind that came from the ground or that grazed from the ground and not from a laboratory, a factory, or a factory farm. You'll consume better and more vital nutrients to keep your energy moving, and you'll shed your desire for junk food. Avoiding the unnecessary ingredients that they contain will teach your body to stop trying to process them - which it can't do anyway - and you will train your body to focus its energy on metabolizing the natural nutrients you need. Any leftover energy is yours to do with as you please!

Focus On Health, Not Weight

People like to make grandiose statements about dropping a dress size or losing a certain number of pounds. It's a way of attaching a number to their accomplishments, and it helps to indicate progress. While the intention is good, focusing on weights or sizes often means a life of deprivation rather than celebration. Depriving yourself of good healthy meals is not sustainable. It ultimately leads to poor results and a disappointing failure to achieve your long-term goals. If you maintain your focus on keeping up your health, your goals will shift more along the lines of increased energy or feeling happier. When you look at your body from a place of healing, weight loss may result as another happy side effect of resolving your physical symptoms, rather than it being the driving force. Healthy is the new thin.

Remain Mindful

If you've just eaten and still feel hungry, yet you know you're not hungry, it's not food your mind is wanting. It's never about the food, and it never was. Food will never completely satisfy you until you look closely at the associations you have with food, and the stories you make up around food. Sometimes it's the memories of a particular food item, and the experiences around that food that you're trying to recapture. Sometimes it's a belief that eating certain foods, like Hallowe'en candy or Christmas cookies, will bring you back to a happier time in your life. It's a feeling. It's always a feeling. Perhaps it is feelings of belonging, companionship, welcome, acceptance, deserving, or feeling special. Sometimes it is the avoidance of feelings like loneliness, boredom, or distance from others. But it's always a belief that food will either give to you, or relieve you from, these things, these feelings. Be mindful that you cannot return to that wonderful time and place when you were eating cupcakes as a child on a special day. Will another cupcake take you back to that place? You have always treasured food as a gateway to your feelings. It's time you started to treasure your self, and leave out the middle-man.

Move More

Your lymphatic system is your body's janitorial service, and it's an essential part of your autoimmune system. This system doesn't have a central pump, as the circulatory system has the heart, and so it relies on body movement in order to move impurities out of your body efficiently. You have over six hundred lymph nodes throughout your body, and the first thing in the morning is one of the best times to get them all moving (mostly because you've been relatively still for several hours). You can dance, go out for a run, skip rope, jump on a trampoline, or just do the leg-stretchies and toe-touchies that they taught you in P.E. class all those years ago. We are becoming an increasingly sedentary society, and so keeping your body moving helps to open elimination pathways and restore an enhanced immune system. It will also wake you up in ways that coffee alone cannot, by stimulating your adrenals into cortisol production. The simple act of increased physical motion will help keep you feeling alert throughout your day. So if you're the type whose first agenda item every morning is to shuffle into the kitchen and forage for coffee, consider whether it's much of a change for you to incorporate some form of physical activity while you're waiting for the coffeepot. You will begin to feel a difference rather quickly. Start with small goals, develop them into a daily routine, and when they start to get easy you can extend them bit by bit.

Remember To Breathe

If there is one simple thing you can easily learn to do, it's the habit of regularly taking long deep breaths. Do you really believe that someone needs to remind you to breathe? You breathe all the time, but seldom do we take a moment, close our eyes, and just focus on taking long deep breaths. Breathing deeply from the diaphragm activates the parasympathetic side of the autonomic nervous system, which prepares our bodies to go into "rest and digest" mode. This is essential not only for good digestion, but for proper immune function, restful sleeping and a better mood. It communicates to every cell in your body that you are safe, and we are unable to access this part of our nervous system by just our thoughts. We can only get there by being still and quiet for a few minutes as we focus on our breathing. You will be amazed at what your body can do if you simply allow yourself a few minutes each day to assure your self that life is good and you are OK.

Spend More Time With Nature

I am a self-identified city boy, but I live near a large park in my town that helps me to take a break from things like writing a book and just escape for a few minutes. Living in the Pacific Northwest, there is no end of unspoiled beauty within just a short drive from my home. Being in nature can do wonderful things for one's soul. Even after just a few minutes, the majesty of nature can nourish and restore you in ways that nothing man-made can do. As you walk, take the time to experience the various ways in which nature constantly creates and rebuilds itself. This is something that you can easily use to generate creative and restorative energy within your self. The inspiration and empowerment you receive from this will help you to understand that each of us is just a part of something much greater than ourselves.

Maintain An Attitude of Gratitude

Changing how you feel sometimes requires creating an entirely new perspective on how you look at life. That level of change starts out well if you become aware to all that you have, and become sincerely thankful for it. Create your own gratitude list, either in your mind or on paper, and make it your daily habit to review it. You are alive which means you have your health, you cast a shadow which means you are in the sunshine, you have dishes to wash which means you have food and the money to pay for it, you have huge piles of laundry to do because you have people in your life to care for (even if it's only you), and so on. You can start with little things, and soon you'll end up with a limitless list of all the things for which to be grateful. Gratitude is the perfect antidote for dissatisfaction and resentment.

Find Your Passion

Create a list of things that you love doing, and then start doing more of them. There are no limits to what you can put on your list, big things or small, and you will soon find that where your mind goes, your energy follows. Putting energy behind making a list like this will create energy around the things on the list, and that energy will begin to build until your passion becomes something that you just naturally do. Some of us have gotten so far out of touch with our passions, with what makes us feel good, and with the things that serve our health and our spirit. Creating a list lets you recognize the things that make you feel the most energy. If you look back at your list several weeks or months or years later and examine all the things that you listed that you never got around to, don't be discouraged. Perhaps the timing wasn't right, or maybe your energy went in another direction after you wrote the list. You will find that reviewing your list frequently, adding new things and crossing off others, renews and refreshes your passion and helps build momentum and growth in your passionate energy. Knowing what your true passions are and actively pursuing them will help you create more happiness in your life and displace negative energy that holds you down. When you are happier, the transitive properties of your energy will cause it to spill out to others around you.

Live Within A Kind Heart

Everyone knows someone who exudes kindness to everyone they meet. Be that person, today and forever. Do all that you can to approach every situation with kindness, grace, and compassion to others. Go beyond what you think is enough. Give kindness your all. When something upsets you or makes you angry, however slightly, you can teach yourself to take a moment and not react to it. Just observe without judgment. Did that person cut you off in traffic because they are arrogantly self-absorbed, or because they are rushing to take someone to the hospital? Everyone has their own internal struggle and their own story, and if we replace that with our stories and judgments, then we negate them as a person. Even just smiling at passing strangers and acknowledging their presence will brighten up their day and propel your energy forward in a positive direction, and you will create a ripple effect of kindness that spreads out into the world.

Be Beautiful

Beauty is being the best that you can be, inside and out, without the external judgments from others. Being a beautiful, energetic, creative, and helpful spirit is contagious. The energy coming from your own inner beauty radiates from your heart and mind and spreads among everyone you encounter. Consider the fellow I mentioned earlier who looked in his mirror every morning and said, "I love you." Wow! What an empowering way to begin your day! I've adopted that habit for myself, and I hope that you will too. You'll find that it not only improves your attitude for the day but will make you shine from the inside out. If other people are a mirror of your own energy, wouldn't you rather that the people you meet reflect your inner beauty and grace?

Staying Healthy For Life

By now you have been exposed to the basics of creating optimal health for your self. You've learned much about what, how, when, where and why to eat, and you've even begun to tailor that knowledge to fit within your own needs. If it's all gone well, you've begun to change your lifestyle to accommodate what you've found that works better for you. You've developed new tastes and begun new habits, and more importantly you are opening up to creating a new way of life for your self in which you can move beyond your greatest expectations.

Now you are ready to move forward into a new life that you've designed and created for your self. Your old ways of living are becoming less appealing and more distant. You've begun to notice palpable differences, however slight, in how you view the world and your place in it. Most importantly, you realize that you now have limitless possibilities, and you can choose any of them to follow, or you can follow several at once. You know and feel more, and you can accept more and newer things as they approach you. You move closer and closer to living the promise of self-mastery.

Living Within Change

The most difficult part of changing any new behavior is in getting started. It takes quite a lot of motivation to head to the gym for a workout after an exhausting day at work, but once you

123

actually begin the workout it doesn't take as much motivation to finish it. Once you've started going twice a week, it doesn't take much more effort to start going three times a week, then four and five and so on. For this reason, one of the best things you can do for building a new behavior is to start with a remarkably small habit. As Leo Babauta, creator of the Zen Habits web site, says, "Make it so easy you can't say no."

New habits should come to you as simple and non-threatening. Start with a behavior that is so small it seems easy and reasonable to do it each day. If you set a goal to be able to do a hundred push-ups every day, could you start by doing ten? If you would like to read more books, read just a page or two every night until you find you can't get to sleep without reading a little more before turning in. You may sit staring at your list of New Year resolutions and quickly become overwhelmed by the length and gravity of your desire to create change. You might go through and begin cherry-picking some of the easier ones to take on first, and this is actually a great idea. It's like rocking the car to break its inertia, after which pushing the car is not so difficult. Start with gentle pushes and you will find yourself smoothly rolling along soon enough.

Focus on changing your behavior, not on the outcome. Nearly every conversation about goals and resolutions rests its focus on the result. How many dress sizes do you want to lose? How quickly do you want to resolve your diabetes? We are naturally outcome-based because we want to be able to measure the results of our new behaviors. The problem with this is that creating new goals won't deliver new results; only new lifestyles do. Changing your lifestyle is a process, not an event, and for this reason you should focus your energy and awareness to creating a new lifestyle so that you will naturally come to a new result set.

Sometimes creating change involves creating a whole new environment for your self. Creating positive new habits is impossible in an environment of negativity. Just try eating more healthy food when you are surrounded by nothing but fast-food chains; try keeping focused on positive thoughts when your work environment is rife with negativity; or try focusing on the task at hand when you are assaulted with random calls, text messages, emails and other distractions. We find it difficult to face the fact that our behavior is based on a reaction to external stimuli. In fact, the lifestyle you have been living has a direct correlation to the environment in which you spend most of your time. The single greatest factor in facilitating change in your life is to create an environment that is designed to help you succeed.

Here's a simple example: You wake up to an alarm clock every morning, and the first thing you do is pick up your phone that's been charging on the nightstand, conveniently in reach of your bed. You start your day by checking for emails, reading updates on Facebook and Twitter and other social media, and perhaps scanning news headlines and checking the weather for the new day. By the time you get up and on your feet, you have been bombarded by a few dozen new distractions that are now occupying your thoughts. You might have responded or reacted to a few of them, or maybe you are thinking of how you might respond to them later. Already your mind is swirling with so many new pieces of information that take up precious thought cycles, and you haven't even gotten dressed yet.

If this sounds like you, the easiest way to change this behavior is to change your environment. Instead of having your phone by the bed where it is so easy to tend to it during your first waking moments, leave your phone as far away as possible from your bed. If your phone is the cause of this early morning chaos, that's the part of your environment you need to change first. It's a simple change that can make a world of difference to you.

Another simple change is to create a space in which you will be comfortable doing your new morning routine. Get up and stretch, start doing a few simple exercises, write in a journal or just lie in bed and do some deep breathing meditations. If your environment doesn't change, you can't expect to create change in your self. By changing your environment, you will have already started creating the change you need in your life.

Always remember that small changes add up. Whenever people talk about their goals, they tend to describe the minimum they'd like to achieve. They may want to read a new book every week or put aside five thousand dollars each year or lose twenty pounds by swimsuit season. If the underlying assumption is that your goals need to be big in order to matter, you will surely meet with disappointment if you don't reach your 100% mark. By repeating patterns of small changes in your behavior, you will chip away at your goal and create healthier new habits that will get you to your goal surely and steadily. Instead of striving to attain the 100% mark all at once, which is rather unrealistic, try pushing into ten percent now, and another ten percent later, and so on. If it starts to feel like it's becoming easier, that shows you that you can push it just a little more each time.

Exercise For Life

As most people know, diet and exercise are the two primary pathways to a healthier life. Too many people these days forego both of them, but the ones who want to become healthy will make their first move in the direction of the local gym. They will spring for the annual membership, hire a personal trainer, spend hours each day sweating to loud workout music, and ultimately achieve little of the results they'd hoped for. The results that most people are looking for is weight loss, a slimmer figure, or even spot reduction, but exercise is only part of the equation.

In talking to several personal trainers that I know, they tend to agree that nutrition is more than half of the equation. If you spend half an hour on a treadmill, an elliptical, or a stair machine, you will burn off about 610 calories (assuming a 205 lb. male running an eight-minute mile; your mileage will vary). Then what? You go to dinner after the gym and consume that much or more in empty calories that don't help you get the nutrition you need. You end up with a nutritional deficit, a much longer path to your goal, and a half an hour of your life that you'll never get back.

I am certainly not at all saying that exercise is unimportant; quite the contrary. As I've mentioned, daily exercise is crucial in maintaining good physical condition, and vigorous exercise can help your body do amazing things. Without the proper nutrition to support it, though, your performance goals at the gym will come to you more slowly. This can end up in frustration to the point of wanting to give up and go back to the sofa with a tub of ice cream, assured that you are doomed to the shape and size that you are. By golly, you tried, but it just didn't seem to work for you because somehow you're different. The real issue is that you tried, yes, by diligently going to the gym more than you used to, but without proper nutritional support, your efforts ultimately fell short of your goals.

With that said, the benefits of regular exercise are clear. Sometimes a walk around the block after dinner isn't enough, but at least it's a start. Once you begin the habit of walking around the block after dinner, you can easily move up to walking around two blocks, and three, and then more until you can start to run. You may also get to meet more of your neighbors that way. Running in the morning seems to work best for most people, but exercise however you want and whenever you want. When a certain exercise starts to seem easy to you, it means that you can push it just a little further, and you will soon be amazed at how quickly you've begun to improve. The point is to keep pushing yourself to your limits and a bit beyond - not so much that you end up with an injury, mind you, but your body can take more than you might imagine. And the benefits are immense.

Regular exercise can single-handedly lower HDL levels, the high-density lipoproteins that can contribute to atherosclerosis and other cardiovascular conditions. Strenuous exercise, less like a walk around the block and more like the Ironman Decathlon, has been shown to actually restore damaged intestinal villi, the magic fingers in your intestinal lining that absorb nutrients from your food[11]. Furthermore, researchers have found that a sedentary life can be more harmful than obesity, and that regular exercise can lower your chances of an early death by up to 30%.[12]

I've never known someone who is so busy that they can't find a half an hour three times a week to exercise. Give up a TV show, stop checking social media for a while, pretend you haven't got a job or other responsibilities for just a half hour a few times a week. Set aside a daily training time commitment of thirty minutes including warm up and cool down periods, plus brief spurts of three minutes doing some sort of intense exercise. The people who can't find time for this are usually just too lazy or indifferent to want to do it, and I say this with full authority because I was once one of those people.

---

[11] Honestly, though, I've come from a place of severe intestinal damage, and, in the depths of my illness, a hard workout was quite out of the question. Granted.

[12] Ulf Ekelund, Ph.D., senior investigator scientist, Medical Research Council Epidemiology Unit, University of Cambridge, U.K.; David Katz, M.D., M.P.H., director, Yale University Prevention Research Center, New Haven, Conn.; Samantha Heller, M.S., R.D., senior clinical nutritionist, New York University Medical Center, New York City; Jan. 14, 2015, American Journal of Clinical Nutrition

Epilogue

Perhaps the toughest thing about what I do is getting people to change. What we choose to eat is very personal to each of us, and it's one of the two basic survival instincts along with procreation. Eating is just as much a part of self-preservation as running away from a predator. In this case, we are running towards our prey, which might just be a bison or fruit growing from a tree or a sandwich. It's built into our nature, and into the very nature of all living beings. Self-nourishment is self-preservation.

I once knew a guy whose job had him traveling around the world; six weeks in Mexico City, a month in Stockholm, and so on. He would only eat at McDonalds, and he told me that it was the only way he knew he was getting something he would like. He might have been inwardly averse to eating something he might not like, and that his world would somehow fall apart because of that experience. I used to travel quite a bit in my former career, too, and I remember spending a week doing business in Osaka and Tokyo. I ate a lot of questionable things like sashimi-grade chicken and tempura king crab legs, fried shell and all, but I'd never say I had a bad meal.

Change is an inevitable force. The universe is constantly changing around us, even when we think there's nothing happening. Resistance to change comes from wanting to hold onto a past that has already left us, and from facing a future that seems uncertain. We feel that it is all uncontrollable, or that somehow we must exert control over other things, people and situations in our lives. Control is illusory and fleeting. Yet we can shape our own future somewhat. We can influence the directions that we plan for our lives such that, when the unexpected sideswipes us, we can still reasonably expect that we will not veer too far off our intended path.

As I was writing this book, I often solicited the opinions of my friends for guidance, and many of their thoughts and suggestions have made their way into these pages. Some saw the title as too abrupt. They felt that it was too negative, that I was admonishing them for having a poor outlook on their life and their body, or that it reminds them of something that they are not doing right. It's difficult when we hear someone tell us that our best efforts are not working for us, and yet that's sometimes what we need to hear most. Negativity implies positivity, and vice versa. Until we can be aware to the negative things that control our lives, we can't do anything with the positive things. We can choose instead to live inside a shiny pink bubble where we believe that everything inside is bliss and perfection, ignoring everything that exists outside that bubble. I'm as guilty of spending some quality time inside that bubble as anyone else you could name.

Here's another law of inertia for you, from my father's lips to your ears: "A body at rest tends to remain at rest, and a body in motion tends to remain in motion, unless acted upon by an outside force." It takes an outside force - a friend, a family member, a self-help book - to prick that bubble and expose you to the reality that you can do better. You can begin treating your body like your friend and ally, and you can use to your advantage the knowledge that that alliance brings. I wish you only the best in your journey.

If you live only for a day, or even an hour, you should live for the dreams, values, and spirit you have chosen. Don't live an habitual life, trained to the familiar and the comfortable. Through self-examination and self-challenge, create change and adjust your track toward growth and completion.

Ilchi Lee

Appendix I

Five Steps To Optimal Health

The path to your own personal wellness can be divided into five segments. Naturally, the lines dividing them will blur, but the different stages are clearly defined. These steps derive from ancient Taoist teachings, but if you do not identify as a Taoist, I urge you to view them through the lens of your own form of understanding. In the end, you will have the knowledge, determination, and motivation to be on the path to optimal health and to stay on it for life.

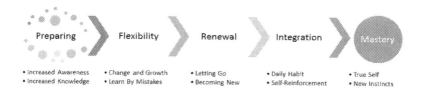

Preparing	Flexibility	Renewal	Integration	Mastery
• Increased Awareness	• Change and Growth	• Letting Go	• Daily Habit	• True Self
• Increased Knowledge	• Learn By Mistakes	• Becoming New	• Self-Reinforcement	• New Instincts

Preparing

The first stage is just seeking basic relief of all your current symptoms. You feel aches, pains, and both physical and emotional stress. You suffer from various diseases and conditions, from small things like dandruff to more serious maladies that cause you considerable concern. It might be that you are unconsciously choosing to hold on to them, and that usually comes from a place of fear. You hang on to past behaviors because they feel comfortable and are hard to let go. I have even heard people make jokes knowing that the food they are eating is bad for them, and they know they are right but something is keeping them in the same patterns. Peer pressure, herd mentality, the unknown - when you unpack these feelings, you find that they are all rooted in feelings of fear. Once you've identified them for what they are, you can begin to examine exactly what it is that you fear the most. Unpacking and examining the fear that prevents you from moving forward is instrumental for beginning the important change you seek to create.

Flexibility

Once you are beginning to feel relief from your symptoms, you can create a clearing for correction and strengthening. You will notice that things are beginning to work better. Your digestion, blood pressure, ability to handle life's stressors, all will be noticeably more efficient and effective. Your energy increases somewhat, and you may even sleep better. You will slow down the momentum of what had been holding you back, and you begin to reverse that energy into a more positive direction. In this clearing you've made, as a result of chasing after and relieving your symptoms, you can continue adding new habits and procedures that are designed to shore up those weaknesses that you had once accepted as the "new normal."

Renewal

You soon find your self in the stage of feeling better, and it's happening more often. It dawns on you that this is how you are now. Energy is at its peak, you sleep well nearly every night and you arise feeling as if you can take on the world. This is the stage that everyone wants; if they could just get to this point it would be enough. Starting to clear away your physical and mental stress is truly liberating, and even better is the feeling that you now have the tools you need to enjoy greater health and self-confidence as your life continues. Surely, at some point you will catch a cold, break a leg, eat something that disagrees with you, and so on. Life will happen to you, in other words. But as you go forward you will carry with you a better understanding of what you can do about these things when they come up in your life.

Integration

This is a stage in which you combine everything you've learned into the way in which you will now manage your life. You enter an area of rehabilitation, detoxification, and restoration that continue to support your life. Your body was not so much designed to be healthy as it was designed to adapt to the world and its many stressors, and by the time you've reached this stage you have become able to identify the various stressors in your life and how you can manage them. You may know, for instance, that eating gluten makes you weak, that dairy products make you gassy, that certain foods agree with you more than others. You've been paying attention and can now see the cause and effect of your food choices. You are making better choices now.

Mastery

At this point you are deep into a life of supportive self-care, as well as being better able to care for those around you. Your kids enjoy better health, your spouse has begun feeling better, and all of your friends look upon you as the go-to for nutritional advice. It's not that you've become some kind of all-knowing perfect being, but you've worked on refining your skills for so long that they are a part of who you are now.

At the outset this process may seem like a difficult challenge to you, but in order to go on this journey you have to take the first step. As you go through this process and adhere to its principles, you will be astounded at what you've done before you are even halfway through. Millions before you have overcome serious diseases and lost literally tons of excess weight by just changing everything about everything they thought they knew about their food. That means that you can do it too, because you are no better or worse than any of them.

There is an often-told parable of two monks, master and student, walking together from one city to the next. Along the way, they come across a rather large river with a strong current. Beside the river sat an old woman who told the travelers that she is too small and frail to cross the river safely on her own. The master picked her up, carried her across the river, and set her down safely on the other side. As they resumed their walk, the younger student was puzzled. As monks, they were proscribed from touching women, and yet the master had blithely picked her up and carried her regardless. The student asked the master why he'd done that, and he got no answer as they continued to walk. Later, just before they got to their destination, the student could not hold his concern any longer and asked again, "Master, you know we're not allowed to touch women. Why did you do that?" The master stopped, turned to his student and replied, "I left that woman by the side of the river. Why are you still carrying her?"

Hearing this story can make you think about the things you are still carrying around with you. Do you ever ask why you are still holding on to things from your past? Do you ever get a reasonable answer? Once you think you have found the answer, disregard your simple explanation and ask again. Keep sweeping away the obvious and asking again and again to dig deeper and find the true meaning behind your actions.

The more you keep asking these questions, and the more you sweep away the obvious answers, the more you will learn about your self and the more you will grow into a life of change. There is nobody else in the world who can do this for you.

Appendix II
Five Mental States

There are five states that you can use to help drive you along on your path to change. Find a balance with them to help create new activities and new ways of thinking, in an effort to guide you into the change that you seek in your life.

Positivity

Approach each thing you do every day with an air of positivity. Act as if everything is going to work out perfectly, no matter what you are doing. Step out of your victim mentality and into one of self-mastery. Repeating positive messages to your self, such as, "I am good at everything I try," "I am a beautiful person," "I have infinite strength and wisdom," "I can create anything," will counteract the messages in your head that repeat statements to the contrary. If it's true that we talk to ourselves more than we talk to anyone else, why not use positive messaging instead of harmful negativity?

Activity

Don't just stand there, do something! You might make embarrassing mistakes, but without some sort of action there can be no progress. People who have accomplished the most throughout history are often the ones who felt they were the least prepared, and as they find themselves thrust into difficult situations they ended up surprising themselves and those around them by their own unique actions and untapped abilities. Counteract the voices in your mind that offer up excuses, reasons, explanations, and justifications. What do you think is the worst that could happen if you just do it?

Gratitude

Be grateful for everything you have, no matter how small. There will always be others who have a better house or car or job or life, but you have what you have and that's something about which you should be supremely grateful. When you wake up in the morning, make a habit of looking directly at your self in the mirror and saying affirming statements that will honor the person that you know you are. When you show gratitude in everything you do, you transcend your ego and get over your self.

Humility

The Latin root word is *humus*, which means earth or soil. When you become humble, you have stepped off your self-made pedestal and stripped away your ego to return to the most basic element from which you came. When you return to your base level of existence, you can rise up to become truly positive, active, grateful and sincere. Humility is a state in which your ego does not exist. It is only from a place of humility that you can start to transcend your ego – to **get over your self** - and begin the transformative process.

Sincerity

None of the above will work if you do not have true sincerity in your heart. All of the thoughts, emotions, feelings, and preconceptions of your past can rob you of your ability to be truly sincere. Learn to let go of cynicism, resignation, and judgment, and become truly authentic in every thought, word, and deed. When you've broken down the walls of your own hollow "reality," you can create a space for a true reality that will become manifest in everything you think and do and say.

Appendix III

Food Cravings

Here is a guideline you can consider whenever you are craving certain foods. It can help satisfy or even prevent those cravings while providing you with a better form of the nutrients that your body has been missing.

If you crave this...	*what you need is...*	*and so you should eat more of these:*
Chocolate	Magnesium	Raw nuts and seeds, legumes, fruits
Sweets	Chromium	Broccoli, grapes, cheese, dried beans, calves liver, chicken
	Carbon	Fresh fruits
	Phosphorus	Chicken, beef, liver, poultry, fish, eggs, dairy, nuts, legumes, grains
	Sulfur	Cranberries, horseradish, cruciferous vegetables, kale, cabbage
	Tryptophan	Cheese, liver, lamb, raisins, sweet potato, spinach
Bread, toast	Nitrogen	High protein foods: fish, meat, nuts, beans
Oily snacks, fatty foods	Calcium	Mustard and turnip greens, broccoli, kale, legumes, cheese, sesame

If you crave this ...	what you need is ...	and so you should eat more of these:
Coffee or tea	Phosphorous	Chicken, beef, liver, poultry, fish, eggs, dairy, nuts, legumes
	Sulfur	Egg yolks, red peppers, muscle protein, garlic, onion, cruciferous vegetables
	NaCl (salt)	Sea salt, apple cider vinegar (on salad)
	Iron	Meat, fish and poultry, seaweed, greens, black cherries
Alcohol	Protein	Meat, poultry, seafood, dairy, nuts
	Avenin	Granola, oatmeal
	Calcium	Mustard and turnip greens, broccoli, kale, legumes, cheese, sesame
	Glutamine	Supplement glutamine powder for withdrawal, raw cabbage juice
	Potassium	Sun-dried black olives, potato peel broth, seaweed, bitter greens
Chewing ice	Iron	Meat, fish, poultry, seaweed, greens, black cherries
Burned food	Carbon	Fresh fruits
Soda and other carbonated drinks	Calcium	Mustard and turnip greens, broccoli, kale, legumes, cheese, sesame
Salty foods	Chloride	Raw goat milk, fish, unrefined sea salt
Acid foods	Magnesium	Raw nuts and seeds, legumes, fruits
Preference for liquids rather than solids	Water	Flavor water with lemon or lime. You need 8 to 10 glasses per day.
Preference for solids rather than liquids	Water	You have been so dehydrated for so long that you have lost your thirst. Flavor water with lemon or lime.

If you crave this ...	what you need is ...	and so you should eat more of these:
Cool drinks	Manganese	Walnuts, almonds, pecans, pineapple, blueberries
Pre-menstrual cravings	Zinc	Red meats (especially organ meats), seafood, leafy vegetables, root vegetables
General overeating	Silicon	Nuts, seeds; avoid refined starches
	Tryptophan	Cheese, liver, lamb, raisins, sweet potato, spinach
	Tyrosine	Vitamin C supplements or orange, green, red fruits and vegetables
Lack of appetite	Vitamin B1	Nuts, seeds, beans, liver and other organ meats
	Vitamin B3	Tuna, halibut, beef, chicken, turkey, pork, seeds and legumes
	Manganese	Walnuts, almonds, pecans, pineapple, blueberries
	Chloride	Raw goat milk, unrefined sea salt
Tobacco	Silicon	Nuts, seeds; avoid refined starches
	Tyrosine	Vitamin C supplements or orange, green and red fruits and vegetables

Eat more of the things from the right-hand column to get the things you need from the center column, and you'll crave fewer of the things in the left-hand column. Of course, following a properly prepared nutrient-dense diet will help keep stave off these cravings from happening as you move forward with your new ways of eating.

Appendix IV

Lists of hidden sugars and carbohydrates

I stated earlier that I want you to become avid readers of product labels. Here's a list that will help you to get sugar out of your diet, as well as the diets of your family and even pets.

- anhydrous dextrose
- brown sugar
- confectioner's powdered sugar
- corn syrup
- corn syrup solids
- dextrose
- fructose
- high-fructose corn syrup (HFCS)
- honey
- invert sugar
- lactose
- malt syrup
- maltose
- maple syrup
- molasses
- nectars (e.g., peach nectar, pear nectar)
- pancake syrup
- raw sugar

- sucrose
- sugar
- white granulated sugar

You may also see other names used for added sugars, such as cane juice, tapioca syrup, evaporated corn sweetener, fruit juice concentrate, crystal dextrose, glucose, liquid fructose, sugar cane juice, and fruit nectar. These are not recognized by the FDA as ingredient names.

Source: USDA web site (http://www.choosemyplate.gov/weight-management-calories/calories/added-sugars.html)

Appendix V
Food Journal

Write down every bite that you eat. Yes, everything. Note the time of day and how you were feeling before, during, and after eating. If you have three cashews, a candy bar, or a cup of tea, write that down as well. Doing this makes you more aware of what you are eating, when you are eating it, what times of day you are eating certain things, and how it affects your mood. There is a "cheat sheet" on page 138 so you can use numbers as a form of shorthand. As you make note of this more and more, you increase your awareness around your relationship to food.

This is something that I regularly ask my clients to provide for me. I would like to see a minimum of three consecutive days to give me a good idea of what they are eating, as well as the how, when, where, and why questions around their food. One client, a construction worker, admitted that one day he and his co-workers just went to the supermarket for lunch and he got some fried chicken. He earned major points with me for his honesty, and that opened up a discussion around why he felt that convenience is more important than his health.

Another thing you can start doing is to take a photo of every meal, drink, or snack that you have. Since most people have smart phones these days, this can build into an easy habit that will keep you more in touch with what you are using to nourish your body. Be as complete as you can with this. If a friend offers half of their cookie to you, just take a photo of your half of it. Sharing this with your healthcare practitioner would also be a good way to earn extra credit.

I hereby give you my permission to make copies of the table on the next page and use it to create your own food journal. It's not something that you'll need to do forever, but once you are in the habit of tracking everything you eat and drink you will begin to notice that you have become more in touch with your body. And that's what this is all about, isn't it?

FOOD JOURNAL			
	Time	What you had	How you felt
Breakfast			
Snack			
Lunch			
Snack			
Dinner			
Snack			

Index

G

GMO 31, 72

H

heartburn 12, 111
Heaton, Ken 16
Herings Law of Cure 111
Hightower, Jim 49
Hitler, Adolf 45
Hollis, James 43
homeostasis 3, 61, 114
hydration 19, 63
hypochlorhydria 12
hypothalamus 3, 55, 86, 90

I

indigestion 12
inflammation xiv, 59
innate intelligence 3
irritable bowel syndrome (IBS) 18

J

Jung, Carl G. 36
junk food 73

L

leptin 56, 90, 95
Lingual-Neural Testing xvi
lipogenesis 66
lymphatic system 14

M

macronutrients 52, 60, 70
minerals 5, 21, 22, 60, 63, 68, 69

N

Nutritional Therapy
    Association xix

P

parasympathetic 87, 119
pH scale 11
phytonutrients 58
Pollan, Michael 69
polysaccharides 5, 10
prostaglandin 59
protein 30, 52, 72, 141, 142

Q

quinoa 72

S

salt 69, 142, 143
serotonin 67
soy 72
Standard American Diet (SAD)
    22, 26, 52, 53
stomach 11, 13, 23, 69, 87, 88,
    96, 111
sugar xvi, 3, 48, 65, 91, 105, 144
    addiction 66
    blood sugar regulation 66
sympathetic 86, 88

U

urine 19

V

vegetarian/vegan diets 71
villi 13
vitamins xvi, 5, 19, 58, 60

W

About the author

Jeff Woiton has been around food most of his life, starting in a hospital kitchen at age 16 and, more recently, running an upscale cafe on a downscale Caribbean island. As a certified Nutritional Therapy Practitioner, he's combining years of experience in culinary arts, restaurant management and helping others in order to create an environment that cares about the client first and foremost. Though most of his career has been in the technology sector, he's recently made a transition into helping people rather than things.

He firmly believes that food is medicine; more specifically, whole, natural foods are essentially medicine and most else is a slow form of poison. In his practice, he seeks to help people undo years of poor eating habits and adopt a new lifestyle that embraces wellness. Jeff recently brought his own battle with Crohn's Disease into complete remission and now feels as though he's in the best health of his life. He's been where you are, and he can show you how to go beyond what you may have learned or believed, and then helps you create a clearing to step into what you can make possible for your self.

Jeff is a member of the Nutritional Therapy Association, the American Nutrition Association, the Price-Pottenger Nutrition Foundation, the Alliance for Natural Health USA, and the Weston A. Price Foundation. He also serves on the board of Washington Action for Safe Water, an anti-fluoridation organization, as their Nutritional Sciences Advisor.

Notes

Printed in the United States
By Bookmasters